Study Guide for

The Anatomy and Physiology Learning System

Third Edition

Edith Applegate, MS

Professor of Science and Mathematics
Kettering College of Medical Arts
Kettering, Ohio

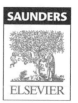

SAUNDERS

ELSEVIER

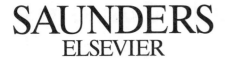

1600 John F. Kennedy Boulevard
Suite 1800
Philadelphia, PA 19103-2899

Study Guide for
The Anatomy and Physiology Learning System

ISBN-13: 978-1-4160-2585-6
ISBN: 1-4160-2585-5

Printed in the United States of America.

Last digit is the print number: 9 8 7 6 5 4 3

Working together to grow
libraries in developing countries

www.elsevier.com | www.bookaid.org | www.sabre.org

ELSEVIER   BOOK AID
            International   Sabre Foundation

Note to Students

Dear Student,

I am excited about Anatomy and Physiology. I find the subject fascinating. I also realize that many students become overwhelmed and frustrated because there is so much to learn, so I have prepared this workbook to help you master, and hopefully enjoy, your study of anatomy and physiology. It contains many tools to help you learn.

Each chapter begins with a list of **key terms, word parts, clinical terms**, and **clinical abbreviations**. These are followed by **objectives/summary** in outline form. **Learning exercises** that have a variety of formats follow the summary. Some are questions to answer or statements to complete. Others are paragraphs in which you fill in missing words, matching exercises, and diagrams to label and color. Many of the exercises ask you to write key words because this helps you learn to spell the words correctly. A small set of colored pencils will be useful because many of the labeling exercises suggest that you color code some of the structures on the diagram.

After the exercises there are **review questions** to lead you through the material again. Now you are ready for the **chapter quiz**. You can use this as a measuring tool to see how well you are doing.

To close each chapter in the workbook, I have prepared some type of word puzzle that relates to the topics in the chapter. These are for those moments when you don't feel like studying and know you should. Maybe the puzzles will get you in the mood. I had a lot of fun preparing the **Fun and Games** pages and I hope you have fun doing them. My philosophy is that you can learn and have fun at the same time.

Carrying this study guide to and from class may help your cardiovascular system, but it won't help you learn anatomy and physiology unless you actually **use** it. You learn better when you are actively involved and this study guide provides a means for your participation in your learning process. It offers another method of study after you have studied your notes and textbook. The study guide also provides a focus for small group study with your peers. Use it. You'll be glad you did.

I hope you enjoy your study of the human body. I would like to hear from you and have your comments and suggestions about ways to improve **The Anatomy and Physiology Learning System**. In closing, I offer my best wishes for success in this course, in your selected curriculum, and in your chosen career.

Sincerely,

Edith Applegate
Professor of Science and Mathematics
Kettering College of Medical Arts

Contents

Chapter 1   Introduction to Anatomy and Physiology 1

Chapter 2   Chemistry, Matter, and Life 17

Chapter 3   Cell Structure and Function 33

Chapter 4   Tissues and Membranes 47

Chapter 5   Integumentary System 63

Chapter 6   Skeletal System 77

Chapter 7   Muscular System 97

Chapter 8   Nervous System 115

Chapter 9   Sensory System 133

Chapter 10   Endocrine System 149

Chapter 11   Blood 165

Chapter 12   Heart 179

Chapter 13   Blood Vessels 193

Chapter 14   Lymphatic System and Body Defense 209

Chapter 15   Respiratory System 223

Chapter 16   Digestive System 239

Chapter 17   Metabolism and Nutrition 257

Chapter 18   Urinary System and Body Fluids 271

Chapter 19   Reproductive System 289

Chapter 20   Development 305

Answers to Learning Exercises 321

Answers to Using Clinical Knowledge 339

1

Introduction to Anatomy and Physiology

KEY TERMS

Anabolism
Anatomical position
Anatomy
Catabolism
Differentiation
Homeostasis
Metabolism
Negative feedback
Physiology

BUILDING VOCABULARY

ab-
ad-
al-
ana-
cardi-
dors-
epi-
gastr-
-graphy
-gram
homeo-
integ-
inter-
intra-
-ism
-itis
-logy
metabol-
path-
pelv-
physi-
proxim-
-scopy
skelet-

-sta-
-tom-
sub-
supra-
vas-
viscer-
-y

CLINICAL TERMS

Acronym
Acute disease
Chronic disease
Diagnosis
Eponym
Prognosis
Remission
Sign
Symptom
Syndrome

CLINICAL ABBREVIATIONS

abd
AE
ant
BK
BP
C
c, cm
cib
DOB
Dx
ENT
F
H&P
lac
N/C

OUTLINE/OBJECTIVES

Anatomy and Physiology

- Define the terms anatomy and physiology and discuss the relationship between the two areas of study.
  - Anatomy is the scientific study of structure.
  - Physiology is the scientific study of function.
  - Anatomy and physiology are interrelated because structure has an effect on function and function influences structure.

Levels of Organization

- List the six levels of organization within the human body.
  - From simplest to most complex, the six levels of organization are chemical, cellular, tissue, organ, body system, and total organism.

Organ Systems

- Name the eleven organ systems of the body and briefly describe the major role of each one.
  - Integumentary system consists of the skin with its derivatives; it covers and protects the body.
  - Skeletal system includes the bones, cartilages, and ligaments; it forms the framework of the body.
  - Muscular system consists of all the muscles in the body; it produces movement and heat.
  - Nervous system includes the brain, spinal cord, and nerves; it receives/transmits stimuli and coordinates body activities.
  - Endocrine system consists of the ductless glands; it regulates metabolic activities.
  - Cardiovascular system includes the blood, heart, and blood vessels; it transports substances throughout the body.
  - Lymphatic system includes lymph, lymphatic vessels, and lymphoid organs; it is a major defense against disease.
  - Digestive system consists of the gastrointestinal tract and accessory organs; it is responsible for the ingestion, digestion, and absorption of food.
  - Respiratory system includes the air passageways and lungs; it is responsible for the exchange of gases between the external environment and the blood.
  - Urinary system consists of the kidneys, urinary bladder, and ducts; it functions to eliminate metabolic wastes from the body.
  - Reproductive system consists of the ovaries and testes with the associated accessory organs; its function is to form new individuals for the continuation of the species.

Life Processes

- List and define ten life processes in the human body.
  - The basic characteristics that distinguish living from non-living forms are organization, metabolism, responsiveness, movement, and reproduction. Advanced life forms, such as humans, have additional characteristics such as growth, development, digestion, respiration, and excretion.
- List five physical environmental factors necessary for survival of the individual.
  - Physical factors from the environment that are necessary for human life include water, oxygen, nutrients, heat, and pressure.

Homeostasis

- Discuss the concept of homeostasis.
    — Homeostasis refers to a constant internal environment.
    — A lack of homeostasis leads to illness or disease.
    — All organ systems of the body, under direction from the nervous and endocrine systems, work together to maintain homeostasis.
- Distinguish between negative feedback mechanisms and positive feedback mechanisms.
    — Homeostasis is usually maintained by negative feedback mechanisms, which inhibit changes.
    — Positive feedback mechanisms are stimulating and cause a process or change to occur at faster rates leading to a culminating event.

Anatomical Terms

- Describe the four criteria that are used to describe the anatomic position.
    — The body is erect, feet are flat on the floor and facing forward, arms are at the sides, and palms and toes are directed forward.
- Use anatomical terms to describe body planes, body regions, and relative positions.
    — Six pair of opposite terms are used to describe the relative position of one body part to another: superior/inferior, anterior/posterior, medial/lateral, proximal/distal, superficial/deep, visceral/parietal.
    — A sagittal plane divides the body into right and left parts; a transverse, or horizontal, plane divides it into upper and lower regions; a frontal, or coronal, plane divides it into front and back portions.
    — The axial portion of the body consists of the head, neck, and trunk; the appendicular portion consists of the limbs or appendages; and specific anatomical terms are used to designate body regions.
- Distinguish between the dorsal body cavity and the ventral body cavity, and list the subdivisions of each one.
    — The dorsal body cavity consists of the cranial cavity, which contains the brain, and the spinal cavity, which contains the spinal cord.
    — The ventral body cavity is subdivided into the thoracic cavity, which contains the heart and lungs, and the abdominopelvic cavity, which contains the digestive, urinary, and reproductive organs.
    — A convenient and commonly used method divides the abdominopelvic cavity into nine regions: epigastric, umbilical, hypogastric, right and left hypochondriac, right and left lumbar, and right and left iliac.

Concepts of Terminology

- Identify the three main parts of words in scientific/medical terminology.
    — The root is the main part or subject of a word.
    — The prefix is placed before a root to alter or modify the meaning of the root.
    — A suffix is attached to the end of a root to modify the meaning of the root.
- Separate words into their component parts to derive their meaning.

LEARNING EXERCISES

Anatomy and Physiology

1. The study of morphology or structure of organisms is called _____.

2. _____ is the scientific study of body functions.

3. Anatomy and physiology are interrelated because the structure of a body part influences its _____ and function has an effect on _____.

4. Identify the specialty areas of anatomy and physiology that are described below by writing the name of the specialty area on the line preceding the description.

_____ Study of external features

_____ Study of cellular structure

_____ Study of prenatal development

_____ Study of the body's defense against disease

_____ Study of drug action in the body

_____ Study of structural and functional changes associated with disease

Levels of Organization

1. The six levels of organization in the body, in sequence from the simplest to the most complex, are _____, _____, _____, _____, _____, _____.

2. The basic living unit of all organisms is the _____.

3. A _____ is a collection of cells with similar structure and function.

Organ Systems

Write the name of the organ system that corresponds to each of the descriptions.

Cardiovascular   Lymphatic   Respiratory
Digestive   Muscular   Skeletal
Endocrine   Nervous   Urinary
Integumentary   Reproductive

1. _____ Consists of the skin, hair, and sweat glands

2. _____ Bones and ligaments

3. _____ Processes food into usable molecules

4. _____   Trachea, bronchi, and lungs

5. _____   Removes nitrogenous wastes from the blood

6. _____   Glands that secrete hormones

7. _____   Cleanses lymph and returns it to the blood

8. _____   Brain, spinal cord, nerves, and sense receptors

9. _____   Blood, heart, and blood vessels

10. _____   Part of the body's defense system

11. _____   Esophagus, stomach, liver, and pancreas

12. _____   Transmits impulses to coordinate body activities

13. _____   Chemical messengers that regulate body activities

14. _____   Transports nutrients, hormones, and oxygen

15. _____   Regulates fluid and chemical content of the body

16. _____   Produces movement and maintains posture

17. _____   Tonsils, spleen, lymph nodes, and thymus

18. _____   Protective covering of the body

19. _____   Forms the framework of the body

20. _____   Ovaries and testes

Life Processes

1. List ten life processes that distinguish living organisms from non-living forms.

2. _____ is the phase of metabolism in which complex substances are broken down into simpler ones.

3. Define anabolism.

4. List five physical factors from the environment that are essential to human life.

Homeostasis

Write the term that is defined by each of the following phrases.

1. _____ Maintenance of a relatively stable internal environment

2. _____ Any condition that disrupts homeostasis

3. _____ Action that has an effect opposite to a deviation from normal; action to maintain homeostasis

4. _____ Mechanisms that stimulate or amplify changes

Anatomical Terms

1. Describe the anatomical position by stating the position of each of the following parts:

   Body is _____

   Face is _____

   Arms are _____

   Palms are _____

   Feet and toes are _____

2. Provide the directional term that correctly completes each statement.

   The nose is _____ to the mouth.

   The elbow is _____ to the wrist.

   Muscles are _____ to the skin.

   The heart is _____, or in front of, the vertebral column.

   The _____ pericardium covers the heart.

3. Name the plane that:

   _____ Divides the body into right and left halves.

   _____ Divides the body into superior and inferior portions.

   _____ Divides the body into anterior and posterior portions.

   _____ Divides the body into right and left portions.

4. Name the most specific body cavity that is described by each of the following phrases:

   _____ Contains the cranial and spinal cavities.

_____   Contains the thoracic and abdominopelvic cavities.

_____   Contains the brain.

_____   Contains the heart and lungs.

_____   Contains the liver, stomach, and spleen.

_____   Contains the spinal cord.

_____   Contains the urinary bladder and rectum.

5. Label the nine regions of the abdomen indicated on the following diagram.

    A. _____

    B. _____

    C. _____

    D. _____

    E. _____

    F. _____

    G. _____

    H. _____

    I. _____

A	D	F
G	B	E
I	H	C

6. Label the body regions indicated in the following figures.

    A. _____

    B. _____

    C. _____

    D. _____

    E. _____

    F. _____

    G. _____

    H. _____

    I. _____

    J. _____

K. _____

L. _____

M. _____

N. _____

O. _____

P. _____

Q. _____

R. _____

S. _____

T. _____

Concepts of Terminology

1. Name the three main parts of a word in scientific terminology. Place a 1 before the part that is first in the word, a 2 before the second part, and a 3 before the last part.

   _____ _____ _____

2. What is the root in the word *gastritis* and what is the meaning of the root?

3. Separate the word *skeletal* into its component parts, give the meaning of each part, and state whether that part is a prefix, root, or suffix.

REVIEW QUESTIONS

1. What is the relationship between anatomy and physiology?

2. Starting with the simplest or smallest level, name in sequence the six levels of organization in the human body.

3. List the eleven organ systems in the body and describe the general functions of each one.

4. What are five characteristics that distinguish living from non-living forms?

5. What are five characteristics that distinguish advanced life forms, such as humans, from other living forms?

6. Name five environmental factors that are necessary to maintain human life.

7. What is meant by "homeostasis" and how is it maintained?

8. How does positive feedback differ from negative feedback?

9. Describe the position of the head, arms, hands, and feet when the body is in anatomical position.

10. Use the indicated directional terms to write sentences that describe the relative positions of the indicated body parts:

    (a) superior/inferior (mouth and nose)

    (b) anterior/posterior (spinal cord and heart)

    (c) medial/lateral (ears and eyes)

    (d) proximal/distal (elbow and wrist)

    (e) superficial/deep (skin and muscles)

11. How are you dividing the body when you cut on each of the following planes?

    (a) coronal plane

    (b) transverse plane

    (c) sagittal plane

12. What are the two major body cavities and which one is larger?

13. What makes up the axial portion of the body?

14. Use two horizontal and two vertical lines to form a grid (like tic-tac-toe), then identify each of the nine areas of the abdominopelvic region.

15. Use two anatomical terms that pertain to specific regions of the head, the arm, the thorax, the abdomen, and the lower extremity.

16. Using the word parts given in this chapter, write a word that means the process of cutting apart.

CHAPTER QUIZ

1. _____ is the scientific study of how the parts of the body work.

2. The smallest unit of organization that is *living* is (a) chemical; (b) cell; (c) tissue; (d) organ; (e) system.

3. Which of the following does *not* represent a correct grouping of organ system/part of system/function? (a) integumentary/skin/cover and protect; (b) endocrine/ductless glands/regulate metabolic activity; (c) respiratory/lungs/exchange of gases; (d) lymphatic/heart/defense against disease; (e) urinary/kidney/excrete metabolic wastes.

4. The "breaking-down" part of metabolism is called _____.

5. Which of the following correctly lists three physical factors from the environment that are necessary to sustain human life? (a) oxygen, metabolism, respiration; (b) water, organization, excretion; (c) oxygen, water, anabolism; (d) oxygen, water, pressure; (e) reproduction, respiration, nutrients.

6. Which one of the following does *not* pertain to a negative feedback mechanism? (a) helps to maintain homeostasis; (b) when blood pressure decreases, the heart beats faster to increase blood pressure; (c) responsible for increased sweating when air temperature is higher than body temperature; (d) when blood sugar level decreases, the hunger center in the brain is stimulated; (e) increases deviations from normal.

7. In anatomical position, (a) your body is erect, arms are behind your back; (b) your eyes are facing the same direction as your palms; (c) you are sitting down with feet forward; (d) feet are forward and palms are in the opposite direction; (e) arms are at your side and palms are facing the opposite direction from your eyes.

8. Which of the following means closer to a point of attachment or origin? (a) superficial; (b) anterior; (c) proximal; (d) medial; (e) superior.

9. The plane that divides the body into anterior and posterior parts is the _____ plane.

10. The region that is in the midline, superior to the umbilical region, is the (a) hypogastric; (b) hypochondriac; (c) lumbar; (d) epigastric; (e) iliac.

11. Place an X before each of the following that pertains to the ventral body cavity.

    _____ Spinal cord

    _____ Heart

    _____ Thoracic cavity

    _____ Small intestines

    _____ Cranial cavity

12. The appendicular portion of the body includes the (a) head and neck; (b) arms and legs; (c) thorax and abdomen; (d) brain and spinal cord; (e) dorsal and ventral cavities.

13. Match the following terms with the appropriate body region.

_____	Skull	A.	antecubital
_____	Buttock region	B.	axillary
_____	Armpit area	C.	cervical
_____	Chest region	D.	cranial
_____	Area behind the knee	E.	gluteal
_____	Middle region of abdomen	F.	oral
_____	Anterior midline of thorax	G.	pectoral
_____	Space in front of the elbow	H.	popliteal
_____	Mouth	I.	sternal
_____	Neck region	J.	umbilical

14. In the word "epicarditis," what is the

    (a) prefix _____

    (b) suffix _____

    (c) root _____

USING CLINICAL KNOWLEDGE

1. Match the definitions on the left with the correct term from the column on the right by placing the corresponding letter in the space before the definition.

     _____ Evidence of disease that can be evaluated or observed by someone other than the patient

     _____ Name of a disease or structure that is based on the name of an individual

     _____ Prediction of the course of a disease and the recovery rate

     _____ A combination of signs and symptoms occurring together that characterize a disease

     _____ Evidence of disease that can only be evaluated by the patient

A. Eponym

B. Prognosis

C. Sign

D. Syndrome

E. Symptom

2. Write the meaning of the following abbreviations.

_____ DOB

_____ H&P

_____ BP

_____ Dx

_____ ac

_____ prn

_____ qid

_____ IV

_____ mg

_____ ant

3. Spelling is important in scientific and medical applications because only one or two incorrect letters may change the meaning. Six of the following words from this chapter are misspelled. Place a check mark (√) in the space before the word if it is spelled correctly. Write the correct spelling in the space if it is spelled incorrectly.

_____ homeostasis

_____ saggital

_____ endocryn

_____ phyziology

_____ epinime

_____ prognosis

_____ limfatic

_____ visceral

_____ hypochondriac

_____ addominopelvic

4. Using word parts from this chapter, write words that have the following meanings.

_____ Pertaining to internal organs

_____ Process of making a recording of the heart

_____ Study of the stomach

_____ Pertaining to the back

_____ Study of disease

FUN AND GAMES

The definitions for 30 words are given on the next page. Determine the correct term for each definition, write the term in the space provided in the word list, then find the terms in the word search puzzle. The word list will be in alphabetical order. Words in the puzzle may be horizontal, vertical, or diagonal and may read forward or backward.

Word Search Puzzle

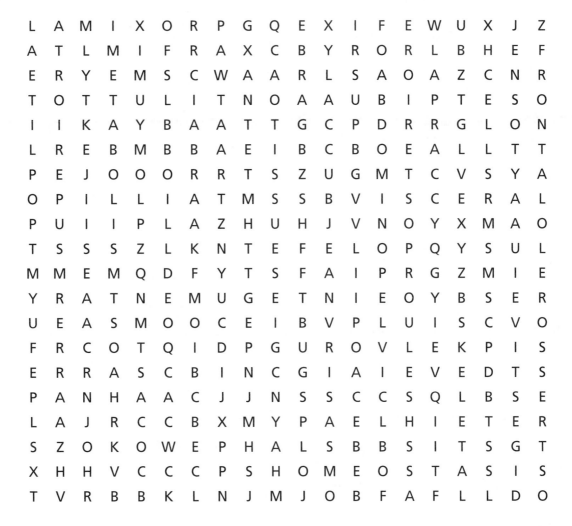

```
L A M I X O R P G Q E X I F E W U X J Z
A T L M I F R A X C B Y R O R L B H E F
E R Y E M S C W A A R L S A O A Z C N R
T O T T U L I T N O A A U B I P T E S O
I I K A Y B A A T T G C P D R R G L O N
L R E B M B B A E I B C B O E A L L T T
P E J O O O R R T S Z U G M T C V S Y A
O P I L L I A T M S S B V I S C E R A L
P U I I P L A Z H U H J V N O Y X M A O
T S S S Z L K N T E F E L O P Q Y S U L
M M E M Q D F Y T S F A I P R G Z M I E
Y R A T N E M U G E T N I E O Y B S E R
U E A S M O O C E I B V P L U I S C V O
F R C O T Q I D P G U R O V L E K P I S
E R R A S C B I N C G I A I E V E D T S
P A N H A A C J J N S S C C S Q L B S E
L A J R C C B X M Y P A E L H I E T E R
S Z O K O W E P H A L S B B S I T S G T
X H H V C C C P S H O M E O S T A S I S
T V R B B K L N J M J O B F A F L L D O
```

Definitions

1. Large ventral body cavity inferior to diaphragm
2. Building phase of metabolism
3. Study of structure
4. Region from elbow to wrist
5. Cheek region
6. Region of the wrist
7. Breaking down phase of metabolism
8. Smallest living unit
9. Body system that includes the esophagus and stomach
10. Thigh region
11. Plane dividing body into anterior and posterior
12. Stable internal environment
13. Body system that includes the skin and sweat glands
14. Toward the side
15. All the chemical reactions that occur in the body
16. Normally maintains homeostasis
17. Lower portion of back of head
18. Study of function
19. Area behind the knee
20. Toward the back, dorsal
21. Closer to the attachment
22. Body system that includes the bronchi and lungs
23. Plane that divides the body into right and left portions
24. System that includes bones
25. A condition that disrupts homeostasis
26. Above another portion
27. Ventral body cavity that contains the heart and lungs
28. Groups of cells with similar structure and function
29. Middle region of abdomen
30. Pertains to the internal organs

Word List

1. _____
2. _____
3. _____
4. _____
5. _____
6. _____
7. _____
8. _____
9. _____
10. _____
11. _____
12. _____
13. _____
14. _____
15. _____
16. _____
17. _____
18. _____
19. _____
20. _____
21. _____
22. _____
23. _____
24. _____
25. _____
26. _____
27. _____
28. _____
29. _____
30. _____

2

Chemistry, Matter, and Life

KEY TERMS

Acid
Atom
Base
Buffer
Carbohydrate
Compound
Covalent bond
Element
Ionic bond
Isotope
Lipid
Molecule
Protein
Radioactive isotope
Solute
Solvent

BUILDING VOCABULARY

aer-
alkal-
carb/o-
bar-
calor-
di-
end-
erg-
-esis
ex-
-genesis
gluc-
hex-
hydro-
-ide
-iform

lact-
lip/o-
-lys
-meter
mono-
-ose
oxy-
pent-
poly-
-ptosis
sacchar-
tetra-
tri-
uni-

CLINICAL TERMS

Endemic
Epidemic
Etiology
Functional disorder
Iatrogenic illness
Idiopathic disorder
Infectious disease
Nosocomial infection
Organic disorder
Pandemic

CLINICAL ABBREVIATIONS

ADL
BRP
CHO
hs
NR
oz

CLINICAL ABBREVIATIONS *(cont'd)*

Px	TO
QOL	UCD
RICE	vs or VS
stat	WA
TBW	

OUTLINE/OBJECTIVES

Elements

- Define matter, element, and atom.
  - Matter is anything that takes up space and has weight.
  - An element is the simplest form of matter.
  - An atom is the smallest unit of an element.
- Use chemical symbols to identify elements.
  - Chemical symbols are abbreviations used to identify elements.

Structure of Atoms

- Illustrate the structure of an atom with a simple diagram showing the protons, neutrons, and electrons.
  - Protons are positively charged particles in the nucleus of an atom and have a mass of 1 amu.
  - Neutrons, also in the nucleus, have the same mass as protons, but have no charge.
  - Electrons are negatively charged particles with negligible mass that are in constant motion in orbits outside the nucleus.
- Distinguish between atomic number and mass number of an element.
  - The atomic number of an element is the number of protons in the nucleus of an atom.
  - The mass number of an element is the number of protons plus the number of neutrons in the nucleus of an atom.
- Describe the electron arrangement that makes an atom most stable.
  - The most stable atoms have eight electrons in their highest energy level or orbit.
- Describe isotopes.
  - An isotope of an element has the same number of protons and electrons, but has a different number of neutrons, which changes the atomic weight.
  - Radioactive isotopes are unstable and emit atomic radiation either in the form of energy or atomic particles.

Chemical Bonds

- Describe the difference among ionic bonds, covalent bonds, and hydrogen bonds.
  - Chemical bonds are forces that hold atoms together.
  - An ion is an atom that has lost or gained one or more electrons; a positively charged ion is a cation; a negatively charged ion is an anion.
  - Ionic bonds are the attraction forces between cations and anions to that form ionic compounds.
  - Covalent bonds result when atoms share electrons; atoms may share more than one pair of electrons, which results in double or triple covalent bonds; an unequal sharing of electrons results in polar covalent bonds.

— Hydrogen bonds are intermolecular bonds, or attractions between molecules, that are formed by the attraction between the electropositive hydrogen end of a polar covalent compound and the negative charges of other molecules or ions.

Compounds and Molecules

- Describe the relationship among atoms, molecules, and compounds and interpret molecular formulas for compounds.
  — Atoms combine in definite ratios to form molecules, which are the smallest units of compounds; the atoms in the molecule are held together by chemical bonds.
  — Molecular formulas use chemical symbols to indicate the types of atoms in a molecule of a compound and numerical subscripts show how many of each atom are present.

Chemical Reactions

- Describe and write chemical equations for four types of chemical reactions and identify the reactants and products in each.
  — Chemical equations are an abbreviated method of showing the reactants and products in a chemical reaction; the reactants are written on the left side of the equation and the products are written on the right side.
  — Synthesis reactions form a complex molecule from two or more simple molecules.
  — Decomposition reactions break down large molecules into simpler ones.
  — In single replacement reactions, an atom in a reactant is replaced by a different atom.
  — Double replacement reactions involve the exchange of two or more elements to form new compounds.
  — Exergonic reactions release energy. Endergonic reactions require energy which is then stored in the chemical bonds.
- Discuss five factors that influence the rate of chemical reactions.
  — The nature of the reacting substances affects the reaction rate.
  — Reaction rates increase as temperature increases.
  — Increasing the concentration of the reactants to an optimum increases the rate of the reaction.
  — Enzymes and other catalysts increase the rate of a reaction.
  — Breaking the reactants into small particles increases the total surface area of the reactants and increases the reaction rate.

Mixtures, Solutions, and Suspensions

- Distinguish among mixtures, solutions, and suspensions.
  — A mixture consists of two or more substances that can be physically separated.
  — Solutions consist of a solute that is being dissolved and a solvent that does the dissolving.
  — In most suspensions, the particles settle if left undisturbed; in colloidal suspensions, the particles are so small they remain suspended but do not dissolve.

Acids, Bases, and Buffers

- Differentiate between acids and bases and discuss how they relate to pH and buffers.
  — Electrolytes form positive and negative ions when they are dissolved in water.

— Acids are proton (hydrogen ion) donors; bases accept protons.
— A pH value indicates the hydrogen ion concentration of a solution; a pH of 7.0 is neutral; acids have a pH less than 7.0; bases have a pH greater than 7.0.
— Neutralization reactions occur between acids and bases to produce salts and water.
— Buffers, which contain a weak acid and a salt of that same acid, resist pH changes by neutralizing the effects of stronger acids and bases.

Organic Compounds

- Describe the five major groups of organic compounds that are important to the human body.
  — Carbohydrates, an important energy source, contain carbon, hydrogen, and oxygen, and include monosaccharides, disaccharides, and polysaccharides; glucose, fructose, and galactose are monosaccharides, or simple sugars, with six carbon atoms, while ribose and deoxyribose have five carbons; sucrose, maltose, and lactose are disaccharides, or double sugars, consisting of two hexose monosaccharides linked together; starch, cellulose, and glycogen are polysaccharides, which consist of long chains of glucose molecules.
  — Proteins are formed from amino acids linked together by peptide bonds; they contain carbon, hydrogen, oxygen, nitrogen, usually sulfur, and often phosphorus.
  — Lipids contain carbon, hydrogen, and oxygen, are insoluble in water, but will dissolve in solvents such as alcohol and ether; the building blocks of triglycerides, commonly known as fats, are glycerol and fatty acids; saturated fats contain only fatty acids that have single bonds between the carbon atoms; phospholipids, which contain phosphates and nitrogen, are important components of cell membranes; steroids are derivatives of lipids and include cholesterol, certain hormones, and vitamin D.
  — Nucleic acids are chains of nucleotides; they contain carbon, hydrogen, oxygen, nitrogen, and phosphorus; DNA is the genetic material of the cell, and RNA functions in the synthesis of proteins within the cell.
  — Adenosine triphosphate (ATP) is a high energy compound that supplies energy in a form that is usable by body cells.

LEARNING EXERCISES

Elements

1. Matter is defined as _____

_____

2. An element is defined as _____

_____

3. Write the chemical symbol for each of the following elements.

_____ Hydrogen   _____ Magnesium   _____ Carbon

_____ Oxygen   _____ Potassium   _____ Phosphorus

4. Identify the element that is represented by each of the following symbols.

_____ Na

_____ Ca

_____ Cl

_____ N

_____ Fe

_____ S

Structure of Atoms

1. Draw a simple diagram that illustrates the structure of an oxygen atom, which has an atomic number = 8 and a mass number = 16.

2. Fill in the information that is missing from the following table.

Particle	Location	Charge	Mass
		0	
			Negligible
Proton			

3. How many protons, neutrons, and electrons are in an atom of potassium, which has an atomic number = 19 and a mass number = 39?

_____ Protons   _____ Neutrons   _____ Electrons

4. The most stable atoms have _____ electrons in their highest energy level.

5. Atoms of a given element that have different atomic weights are called _____.

The difference in atomic weight is due to a difference in the number of _____.

6. Unstable isotopes that emit atomic radiation are called _____.

Chemical Bonds

1. Match each of the following terms with the correct definition below.

   A. ionic bond   D. anion
   B. covalent bond   E. cation
   C. hydrogen bond

   _____   Intermolecular bond

   _____   Ion with a negative charge

   _____   Ion with a positive charge

   _____   Bond between anions and cations

   _____   Bond in which electrons are shared

   _____   Bond between polar covalent molecules

Compounds and Molecules

1. Indicate whether each of the following refers to an atom, a molecule, or a compound.

   _____   Smallest unit of an element that retains the properties of that element

   _____   Formed when two or more atoms are held together by chemical bonds

   _____   Formed when two or more different atoms are chemically combined in a definite ratio

   _____   Smallest unit of a compound that retains the properties of that compound

2. The molecular formula for calcium carbonate, one of the mineral salts in bone, is $CaCO_3$. Name the elements in this compound and tell how many atoms of each element are present.

   _____

   _____

   _____

Chemical Reactions

1. For each example of an equation representing a chemical reaction, indicate whether it is synthesis, decomposition, single replacement, or double replacement and write the formulas for the reactants and products.

Equation: $H_2CO_3 \rightarrow H_2O + CO_2$
                            Carbonic acid

Type of reaction:

Reactants:

Products:

Equation: $N_2 + 3H_2 \rightarrow 2NH_3$

Type of reaction:

Reactants:

Products:

Equation: $MgCl_2 + 2NaOH \rightarrow Mg(OH)_2 + 2NaCl$
                                                              milk of magnesia

Type of reaction:

Reactants:

Products:

Equation: $C_7H_6O_3 + C_2H_4O_2 \rightarrow C_9H_8O_4 + H_2O$
                            salicylic   acetic   aspirin
                              acid   acid

Type of reaction:

Reactants:

Products:

2. In _____ reactions, there is more energy stored in the reactants than in the products. Energy is released in these reactions. Reactions that need an input of energy are called _____ reactions.

3. For each of the following changes, indicate whether the reaction rate will increase (I) or decrease (D).

_____ Grind up the reactants

_____ Add a catalyst

_____ Use more concentrated solutions

_____ Dilute one reactant

_____ Cool the reaction mixture

_____ Increase the temperature

4. What is the meaning of the double arrow in the following equation?

$$CO_2 \;+\; H_2O \;\rightleftharpoons\; H^+ \;+\; HCO_3^-$$

Mixtures, Solutions, and Suspensions

1. When salt is dissolved in water, the water is called the (a) solution; (b) solute; (c) solvent; (d) liquid; (e) dialysate.

2. Solutions (a) are clear; (b) have a fixed composition; (c) settle when left standing; (d) must be separated by chemical means.

3. Indicate whether each of the following combinations is most accurately described as a mixture, solution, or suspension.

_____ Sugar and salt

_____ Blood cells and plasma

_____ Sugar and water

_____ Cytoplasm of the cell

_____ Sand and water

Acids, Bases, and Buffers

1. Substances that form ions in solution are called _____.

2. Indicate whether each of the following phrases refers to an acid or to a base.

_____ Accepts hydrogen ions

_____ Reacts with a buffer to form a weak acid

_____ Has a sour taste

_____ Reacts with OH^- ions to form water

_____ Has a pH of 3.5

_____ Has a slippery, soapy feeling

_____ Donates protons

_____ Has a pH of 8.7

3. Acetic acid ($HC_2H_3O_2$) and sodium acetate ($NaC_2H_3O_2$) are members of a buffer pair.

Which member of the buffer pair reacts to neutralize sodium hydroxide (NaOH) and what neutral product is formed?

Which member of the buffer pair reacts to neutralize hydrochloric acid (HCl) and what neutral product is formed?

Organic Compounds

1. Carbohydrates contain the elements _____, _____, and _____.

2. Three important hexose monosaccharides are _____, _____, and _____.

3. When two monosaccharides are joined by chemical bonds, the resulting molecule is called a _____.

4. Starch, cellulose, and glycogen are examples of a group of carbohydrates called _____.

5. Write the term that is described by each of the following phrases.

_____ Element, in addition to C, H, and O, found in all proteins

_____ Building blocks of proteins

_____ Amino acids that cannot be synthesized in the body

6. Name the following items that pertain to lipids.

_____ The building blocks of triglycerides

_____ Fatty acids that contain all single covalent bonds

_____ Lipids that are an important component of cell membranes

7. Write the term that matches each of the following phrases in the spaces at the left.

_____ Forms the genetic material of the cell

_____ Single-stranded nucleic acid involved in protein synthesis

_____ Building units of nucleic acids

_____ Sugar in DNA molecules

_____ Double-stranded nucleic acids

_____ Five elements in nucleic acids

_____ Nucleic acid that contains uracil

_____ High-energy compound; contains three phosphate groups

8. Match the following substances with the correct class of organic compounds.

A. carbohydrates   B. lipids   C. proteins   D. nucleic acids

_____   Glucose   _____   Glycogen

_____   Amino acids   _____   Hemoglobin

_____   Steroids   _____   RNA

_____   Nucleotides   _____   Disaccharides

_____   Glycerol   _____   Triglycerides

REVIEW QUESTIONS

1. What is matter?

2. What is the simplest form of matter?

3. What is the chemical symbol for (a) oxygen; (b) nitrogen; (c) calcium; (d) potassium; (e) sodium; (f) iron?

4. What component of an atom has
    (a) a neutral charge?
    (b) a negative charge?
    (c) negligible mass?
    (d) a positive charge?
    (e) a mass of one unit?

5. Draw a simplified diagram of a neutral atom that has 11 protons and 12 neutrons.

6. If an atom has 17 protons and 18 neutrons,
    (a) what is the mass number?
    (b) what is the atomic number?

7. How many electrons are in the highest energy level of the most stable atoms?

8. How does an isotope differ from other atoms of the same element?

9. What is the difference between an ionic bond and a covalent bond?

10. What are cations and anions?

11. What is a compound and what is the smallest unit of a compound?

12. The molecular formula for sodium bicarbonate is $NaHCO_3$.
    (a) What elements are in this compound?
    (b) How many atoms of each element are present?

13. Given the following equation:

    $$C_6H_{12}O_6 \ + \ 6O_2 \ \rightarrow \ 6CO_2 \ + \ 6H_2O$$

    (a) What are the reactants?
    (b) What are the products?

14. Identify the type of reaction that is represented by each of the following equations:

    (a) $S \ + \ O_2 \ \rightarrow \ SO_2$

    (b) $Zn \ + \ CuSO_4 \ \rightarrow \ ZnSO_4 \ + \ Cu$

    (c) $2NaClO_3 \ \rightarrow \ 2NaCl \ + \ 3O_2$

    (d) $HgCl_2 \ + \ H_2S \ \rightarrow \ HgS \ + \ 2HCl$

15. Is the following reaction exergonic or endergonic?

    $$ATP \ \rightarrow \ ADP \ + \ P \ + \ energy$$

16. A chemical reaction is proceeding very slowly. Suggest four things you might try to speed up the reaction.

17. The following reaction is reversible.

    $$CO_2 \ + \ H_2O \ \rightleftharpoons \ H^+ \ + \ HCO_3^-$$

    As you breathe, you exhale CO_2 and remove it from the body. What effect does this have on the above reaction? Does the reaction proceed to the right or to the left as a result of exhaling CO_2?

18. What is the difference between a compound and a mixture?

19. What is the difference between a solution and a suspension?

20. What is an electrolyte? Name two common tests (or graphic tracings) based on electrolyte activity in the body.

21. What is the difference between an acid and a base?

22. What are the reactants and products in a neutralization reaction?

23. What is the pH range of acids? of bases?

24. What are the two components of a buffer solution and what is their purpose?

25. List the five major types of organic compounds that are important in the human body.

26. Give examples and state the importance of three hexose monosaccharides, three disaccharides, and three polysaccharides.

27. Describe the structure of proteins.

28. Describe the structure of triglycerides. What is the difference between saturated and unsaturated triglycerides?

29. How do phospholipids and steroids differ from triglycerides?

30. What are three structural differences between the two types of nucleic acids?

CHAPTER QUIZ

1. Write the name of the element represented by each of the following symbols:

    (a) C _____   (c) Cl _____   (e) Cu _____

    (b) P _____   (d) Fe _____   (f) O _____

2. A certain neutral atom has a mass number of 35 and has 17 electrons.

    (a) What is the atomic number of this atom?

    (b) How many neutrons are there in the atom?

    (c) How many protons are there in the atom?

3. Match the terms on the right with the descriptions and definitions on the left.

    _____ Equals the number of protons plus the   A. atomic number
             number of neutrons

    _____ Contained in shells or energy levels   B. electrons
             surrounding the nucleus

    _____ Number of these particles equals the   C. mass number
             number of electrons in a neutral atom

    _____ Determined by the number of protons in   D. neutrons
             the atom

    _____ Have the same mass as protons   E. protons

4. Given the following reaction:

    $$Zn \;+\; CuSO_4 \;\rightarrow\; ZnSO_4 \;+\; Cu$$

    (a) Name the four elements in this reaction.

    (b) Write the chemical formulas for the reactants.

    (c) How many atoms of oxygen are in the products?

    (d) What type of reaction is this?

5. Indicate whether each of the following pertains to an acid or to a base. Use A = acid and B = base.

    _____ Proton donor   _____ Accepts hydrogen ions

    _____ Accepts protons   _____ Donates hydrogen ions

    _____ pH = 8.2   _____ pH = 2.5

    _____ pH = 6.5

6. Given the following neutralization reaction:

   $NaOH + HCl \rightarrow NaCl + H_2O$

   Identify the acid _____, base _____, and salt _____.

7. Assume that a reaction is proceeding at a given rate. Indicate how each of the following will affect the reaction rate. Use F = faster rate and S = slower rate.

   _____ Remove some of the product

   _____ Add an appropriate catalyst

   _____ Decrease the temperature

   _____ Break the reactants up into smaller particles

   _____ Increase the concentration of the reactants

8. Identify each of the following as a monosaccharide (M), disaccharide (D), or polysaccharide (P).

   _____ Cellulose   _____ Glycogen

   _____ Fructose   _____ Lactose

   _____ Galactose   _____ Maltose

   _____ Glucose   _____ Sucrose

9. Classify each of the following as pertaining to carbohydrates (C), lipids (L), proteins (P), or nucleic acids (N).

   _____ Adenine, cytosine   _____ Nucleotides

   _____ Amino acids   _____ Peptide bonds

   _____ Cholesterol   _____ Starch

   _____ Monosaccharides   _____ Triglycerides

10. Which of the following is *not* true about nucleic acids? (a) DNA consists of two strands; (b) both DNA and RNA contain nucleotides; (c) RNA functions in protein synthesis; (d) both DNA and RNA contain a five-carbon sugar; (e) both DNA and RNA contain the nitrogenous base thymine.

USING CLINICAL KNOWLEDGE

1. Match the definitions on the left with the correct term from the column on the right by placing the corresponding letter in the space before the definition.

_____	Nonproprietary drug name assigned by the USAN council	A. Brand name
_____	Presence of a disease in a given population at all times	B. Chemical name
_____	Study of causes of diseases	C. Compound
_____	Alpha-methyl-4(2 methylpropyl) benzene	D. Endemic
_____	An illness that occurs without any known cause	E. Etiology
_____	Smallest unit is a molecule	F. Generic name
_____	Drug name that is assigned by the manufacturing company	G. Idiopathic
_____	An infection acquired from the place of treatment	H. Nosocomial
_____	The water in a normal saline solution	I. Pandemic
_____	A widespread epidemic; occurs over a large geographical area	J. Solvent

2. Write the meaning of the following abbreviations.

_____ CHO

_____ VS

_____ ADL

_____ stat

_____ Px

3. Spelling is important in scientific and medical applications because only one or two incorrect letters may change the meaning. Three of the following words from this chapter are misspelled. Place a check mark (√) in the space before the word if it is spelled correctly. Write the correct spelling in the space if it is spelled incorrectly.

_____ proteen

_____ asid

_____ covalent

_____ elament

_____ iatrogenic

4. What is the meaning of the root in each of the following words?

_____   calorie

_____   tetrad

_____   aerobic

_____   hydrolysis

_____   pentose

_____   alkalosis

_____   lactose

_____   saccharide

_____   lipectomy

_____   glucose

FUN AND GAMES

Determine the words that fit the clues in the left column, then write the words in the boxes in the right column, one letter per box. The circled letters form a scrambled word or phrase. Unscramble the letters to create the word or phrase that matches the final clue.

A. Smallest unit of a compound

Positively charged subatomic particle

Building block of a protein

Accepts protons

Product in a neutralization reaction

Speeds up a chemical reaction

One of the elements in water

A complex carbohydrate

Final clue: High-energy compound _____

B. An element in water

Sugar in RNA

Element always present in proteins

Group of compounds that includes fats

A base in nucleic acids

Positively charged ion

Negatively charged subatomic particle

Resists change in pH

Fat with three fatty acids

Final Clue: Genetic material of the cell _____

3

Cell Structure and Function

KEY TERMS

Active transport
Cytokinesis
Diffusion
Meiosis
Mitosis
Osmosis
Passive transport
Phagocytosis
Pinocytosis

BUILDING VOCABULARY

ab-
ana-
bio-
-cele
cyt-
dist-
-elle
eti-
extra-
hiat-
hyper-
hypo-
-ic-
intra-
iso-
-osis
-ostomy
-phag-
pharmac-
-phil-
-phob-
pino-
-plasm-

quadr-
-reti-
-som-
sub-
ton-
-ul,-ule
-um

CLINICAL TERMS

Anaplasia
Anomaly
Atrophy
Benign
Carcinogen
Congenital disorder
Cytology
Dysplasia
Genetic disorder
Hyperplasia
Hypertrophy
Malignant
Metaplasia
Metastasis
Necrosis
Neoplasm

CLINICAL ABBREVIATIONS

ABC
BCC
CA, Ca
DNA
ECG, EKG
FH
HR

33

CLINICAL ABBREVIATIONS *(cont'd)*

LBW	OP
MRI	PBI
NB	PET
NPO	RDA

OUTLINE/OBJECTIVES

Structure of the Generalized Cell

- Describe the composition of the cell membrane and list five functions of the proteins in the membrane.
  - A selectively permeable cell membrane separates the extracellular material from the intracellular material.
  - The cell membrane is a double layer of phospholipid molecules with proteins scattered throughout.
  - Proteins in the cell membrane provide structural support, form channels for passage of materials, act as receptor sites, function as carrier molecules, and provide identification markers.
- Describe the composition of the cytoplasm.
  - Cytoplasm, the gel-like fluid inside the cell, is largely water with a variety of solutes and has organelles suspended in it.
- Describe the components of the nucleus and state the function of each one.
  - The nucleus, formed by a nuclear membrane around a fluid nucleoplasm, is the control center of the cell.
  - Threads of chromatin in the nucleus contain DNA, the genetic material of the cell.
  - The nucleolus is a dense region of RNA in the nucleus and is the site of ribosome formation.
- Identify and describe each of the cytoplasmic organelles and state the function of each one.
  - Mitochondria are enclosed by a double membrane and function in the production of ATP.
  - Ribosomes are granules of RNA that function in protein synthesis.
  - Endoplasmic reticulum is a series of membranous channels that function in the transport of molecules; rough endoplasmic reticulum has ribosomes associated with it and transports proteins; smooth endoplasmic reticulum doesn't have ribosomes and it transports certain lipids.
  - Golgi apparatus modifies substances that are produced in other parts of the cell and prepares these products for secretion.
  - Lysosomes contain enzymes that break down substances taken in at the cell membrane; they also destroy cellular debris.
  - Cytoskeleton is formed from microfilaments and microtubules and helps to maintain the shape of the cell.
  - Centrioles are located in the centrosome, a dense region near the nucleus, and function in cell division.
  - Cilia are short, hairlike projections that move substances across the surface of a cell.
  - Flagella are long, threadlike projections that move the cell.

Cell Functions

- Explain how the cell membrane regulates the composition of the cytoplasm.
  - The cell membrane controls the composition of the cytoplasm by regulating movement of substances through the membrane.

- Describe the various mechanisms that result in the transport of substances across the cell membrane.
  - Simple diffusion is the movement of particles from a region of higher concentration to a region of lower concentration; may take place through a permeable membrane.
  - Facilitated diffusion requires a special carrier molecule, but still moves particles down a concentration gradient.
  - Osmosis is the diffusion of solvent or water molecules through a selectively permeable membrane; cells placed in a hypotonic solution will take in water by osmosis and will swell due to the increased intracellular volume; cells placed in a hypertonic solution will lose fluid due to osmosis and will shrink or crenate.
  - Filtration utilizes pressure to push substances through a membrane; pores in the membrane filter determine the size of particles that will pass through it.
  - Active transport moves substances against a concentration gradient, from a region of lower concentration to a region of higher concentration; requires a carrier molecule and uses energy.
  - Endocytosis is a process by which solid particles (phagocytosis) and liquid droplets (pinocytosis) are taken into the cell.
  - Exocytosis moves secretory vesicles from inside the cell to the outside of the cell.
- Name the phases of a typical cell cycle and describe the events that occur in each phase.
  - Somatic cells reproduce by mitosis, which results in two cells identical to the one parent cell.
  - Interphase is the period between successive cell divisions; it is the longest part of the cell cycle.
  - Successive stages of mitosis are prophase, metaphase, anaphase, and telophase; cytokinesis, division of the cytoplasm, occurs during telophase.
  - A tumor, or neoplasm, is the result of uncontrolled mitotic activity.
- Explain how meiosis differs from mitosis.
  - Reproductive cells divide by meiosis.
  - In meiosis, a single parent cell produces four cells, each with one-half the number of chromosomes as the parent cell
- Summarize the process of protein synthesis, including the role of DNA and RNA.
  - DNA in the nucleus directs protein synthesis in the cytoplasm. A gene is the portion of a DNA molecule that controls the synthesis of one specific protein molecule.
  - Protein synthesis utilizes mRNA and tRNA in transcription and translation.
  - During the process of transcription, the genetic code is transferred from DNA to mRNA, which carries the information to the sites of protein synthesis in the cytoplasm.
  - A sequence of three nucleotide bases on mRNA represents a codon that codes for a specific amino acid.
  - Translation is the process of creating a protein in response to mRNA codons.
  - Anticodons on tRNA have bases that are complementary to the codons of mRNA; each tRNA carries its specific amino acid to the developing molecule, pairs with the complementary codon on mRNA to determine the amino acid sequence, and releases the amino acid to the developing protein.

LEARNING EXERCISES

Structure of the Generalized Cell

1. List five functions of the various proteins that are found in the cell membrane.

   (a)

   (b)

   (c)

   (d)

   (e)

2. Identify the parts of the generalized cell in the following diagram by placing the correct letter in the space provided by the listed labels. Then select different colors for each structure and use them to color the coding circles and the corresponding structures in the illustration.

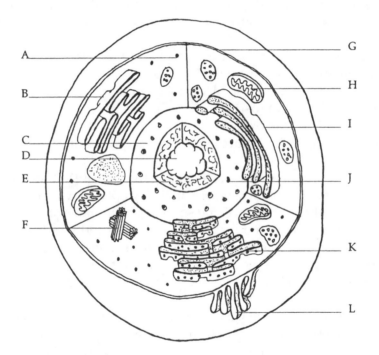

_____ Cell membrane ○	_____ Golgi apparatus ○	_____ Nucleus ○
_____ Centriole ○	_____ Mitochondria ○	_____ Ribosome ○
_____ Chromatin ○	_____ Nuclear pore ○	_____ RER ○
_____ Cilia ○	_____ Nucleolus ○	_____ SER ○

3. Name the cellular component described by each of the following phrases.

_____ Contains enzymes for the production of ATP

_____ Contains digestive enzymes

_____ Prepares products for exocytosis

_____ Granules of RNA in the cytoplasm

_____ Located in the centrosome

_____ Propels substances across the surface of the cell

_____ Membranous transport system within the cell

_____ Long strands of DNA within the nucleus

_____ Functions to move the cell

_____ Dark structure that contains RNA in the nucleus

_____ Semiliquid around the organelles

_____ Controls flow of materials into and out of the cell

_____ Organelle that controls cell functions

_____ Forms the cytoskeleton (2 answers)

_____

Cell Functions

1. Indicate whether each of the following refers to simple diffusion, facilitated diffusion, osmosis, or filtration.

_____ Movement of water through a selectively permeable membrane

_____ Movement of gases in the lungs

_____ Requires a carrier molecule

2. Identify each of the following transport mechanisms as active transport, passive transport, endocytosis, or exocytosis.

_____ Utilizes ATP and a carrier molecule

_____ Phagocytosis

_____ Osmosis

_____ Releases secretory products through the cell membrane

_____ Transports ions from low to high concentrations

_____ Facilitated diffusion

_____ Incorporates fluid droplets into the cytoplasm

3. The accompanying diagram represents two solutions separated by a selectively permeable membrane. Answer the following questions about these solutions.

Solution A	Solution B
5%	1%

Which solution is hypertonic?

Which side will increase in volume because of osmosis?

4. Identify the phase of mitosis that is represented by each of the following illustrations.

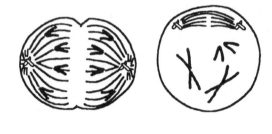 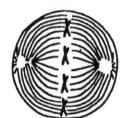

_____ _____ _____

5. Compare mitosis and meiosis by answering the questions in the following table.

	Mitosis	**Meiosis**
In what type of cell does each occur?		
How many new cells are produced in each completed division?		
If the original cell has 46 chromosomes (23 pairs), how many are in each new cell?		

6. A neoplasm develops when _____ is uncontrolled.

7. The following is a sequence of bases in a portion of the gene that codes for the human hormone oxytocin.

A = adenine   C = cytosine   G = guanine   T = thymine   U = uracil

T A C A C A A T G T A A G T T T T G

Write out the sequence of bases on the corresponding mRNA molecule and mark off the codons on this molecule.

Write out the sequence of bases on the six anticodons on the tRNA molecules.

REVIEW QUESTIONS

1. What is a generalized or composite cell?

2. What are the two major types of molecules in the cell membrane? How are they arranged?

3. What are the functions of the proteins in the cell membrane?

4. What is the gel-like fluid inside the cell?

5. Describe chromatin and the nucleolus. Tell where they are located, the major components, and functions of each.

6. What is the structure and function of each of the following cytoplasmic organelles?

   a) mitochondria; b) ribosomes; c) rough endoplasmic reticulum; d) smooth endoplasmic reticulum; e) Golgi apparatus; f) lysosomes

7. What two types of protein structures form the cytoskeleton?

8. Where are the centrioles located and what is their function?

9. What are three differences between cilia and flagella?

10. Label the following diagram of a cell.

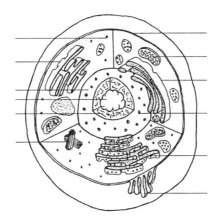

11. What role does the cell membrane have in determining the composition of the cytoplasm?

12. Illustrate the process of diffusion by describing a physiologic example.

13. How is facilitated diffusion different from simple diffusion? In what ways are the two processes alike?

14. Describe the conditions under which osmosis occurs.

15. Describe what will happen to a red blood cell when it is placed in
    (a) an isotonic solution.
    (b) a hypertonic solution.
    (c) a hypotonic solution.

16. Describe the conditions under which filtration occurs.

17. State two ways in which active transport is different from facilitated diffusion. State two ways in which they are similar.

18. What is the difference between endocytosis and exocytosis? What is the difference between phagocytosis and pinocytosis?

19. Describe each of the following:
    (a) interphase
    (b) prophase
    (c) metaphase
    (d) anaphase
    (e) telophase

20. If you start with one cell that has 46 chromosomes,
    (a) how many cells will you have after one complete mitotic division?
    (b) how many chromosomes will be in each cell after mitosis?
    (c) how many cells will you have after one complete division by meiosis?
    (d) how many chromosomes will be in each cell after meiosis?

21. How do neoplasms develop?

22. What are genes and where are they located?

23. What are the complementary base pairs in DNA? What is their role in DNA replication?

24. What is the difference between mRNA and tRNA? What role does each one have in protein synthesis?

25. Transcription and translation both occur in protein synthesis. Describe each of these processes.

CHAPTER QUIZ

1. Match each description with the correct cell component.

   _____ In the cytoplasm; functions in protein synthesis   A. centrioles

   _____ Contains chromatin   B. cilia

   _____ Dense area of RNA in the nucleus   C. endoplasmic reticulum

   _____ Functions in the transport of proteins and lipids   D. flagella

   _____ Protein organelle that functions in cell division   E. Golgi apparatus

   _____ Modifies and prepares substances for secretion   F. lysosomes

   _____ Long, whiplike structures that propel the cell   G. mitochondria

   _____ Contain digestive enzymes   H. nucleolus

   _____ Contain enzymes for making ATP   I. nucleus

   _____ Move substances across the surface of the cell   J. ribosomes

2. Which one of the following does not move solutes from a region of higher concentration to a region of lower concentration? (a) simple diffusion; (b) facilitated diffusion; (c) osmosis

3. Which one of the following uses cellular energy? (a) simple diffusion; (b) active transport; (c) facilitated diffusion; (d) osmosis

4. When a red blood cell is placed in a hypotonic solution, the cell will (a) shrink; (b) swell; (c) crenate; (d) more than one of the responses are correct

5. _____ is described as "cell drinking" because it is taking in liquid droplets.

6. Match the following descriptions with the correct phase of the cell cycle.

   _____ Period of growth and metabolism   A. anaphase

   _____ Chromatin shortens and thickens to form chromosomes   B. interphase

   _____ Chromosomes align themselves along the center of the cell C. metaphase

   _____ Nuclear membrane disappears   D. prophase

   _____ Chromosomes migrate to the end of the cell   E. telophase

   _____ Nucleolus disappears

   _____ Cytokinesis occurs

7. If a cell has 46 chromosomes, (a) there will be 4 cells, each with 23 chromosomes after mitosis; (b) there will be 4 cells, each with 46 chromosomes after mitosis; (c) there will be 2 cells, each with 23 chromosomes after mitosis; (d) there will be 2 cells, each with 46 chromosomes after mitosis.

8. In DNA replication, (a) adenine always pairs with thymine; (b) adenine always pairs with cytosine; (c) adenine always pairs with guanine; (d) cytosine always pairs with thymine; (e) guanine always pairs with thymine.

9. During transcription, (a) DNA is replicated; (b) tRNA transfers an amino acid to a ribosome; (c) a codon on mRNA pairs with an anticodon on tRNA; (d) genetic information is transferred from DNA to mRNA.

10. A sequence of three bases on mRNA is called (a) an anticodon; (b) a gene; (c) an amino acid; (d) a codon; (e) a ribosome.

USING CLINICAL KNOWLEDGE

1. Match the definitions on the left with the correct term from the column on the right by placing the corresponding letter in the space before the definition. Not all terms will be used.

_____ Loss of differentiation of cells; characteristic of cancer	A. Active transport
_____ The route used when administering medications by intravenous, intramuscular, or intradermal injections	B. Anaplasia
	C. Benign
_____ RBCs shrink when placed in a hypertonic solution—an example of this transport process	D. Hyperplasia
	E. Hypertrophy
_____ Enlargement of an organ due to increase in size of constituent cells	F. Meiosis
	G. Mitosis
_____ Process by which a cell may engulf bacteria	H. Necrosis
_____ Death of a group of cells	I. Neoplasm
_____ Any new or abnormal growth; tumor	J. Osmosis
_____ It takes cellular energy to move sodium from low to high concentration in the kidney—an example of this transport process	K. Parenteral
	L. Percutaneous
_____ Not malignant; not recurring	M. Phagocytosis
_____ Type of cell division that produces sperm	N. Pinocytosis

2. Write the meaning of the following abbreviations.

_____ DNA

_____ PBI

_____ LBW

_____ NB

_____ NPO

3. Spelling is important in scientific and medical applications because only one or two incorrect letters may change the meaning. Three of the following words from this chapter are misspelled. Place a check mark (√) in the space before the word if it is spelled correctly. Write the correct spelling in the space if it is spelled incorrectly.

_____ benine

_____ anomoly

_____ meiosis

_____ cytokinesis

_____ displasis

4. Some of the following words may have more than one root. In all cases, give the meaning of the *first* root that appears in the word.

   _____ cytoplasm

   _____ phagocytosis

   _____ hypertonic

   _____ somatic

   _____ reticulum

5. Underline the suffix in each of the following words and write the meaning of the suffix on the line preceding the word.

   _____ hydrophilic

   _____ organelle

   _____ scoliosis

   _____ cellulitis

   _____ pericardial

FUN AND GAMES

1. Structure for cell locomotion
2. Stage when chromosomes are pulled apart during mitosis
3. Base that pairs with adenine
4. Slender rods of protein that are part of cytoskeleton
5. Attracts water
6. Granules of RNA in cytoplasm
7. Same solute strength
8. Division of the cytoplasm
9. Diffusion of solvent through a membrane
10A. Slender threads of DNA and protein in nucleus
10D. Organelle within the centrosome
11. Stage in which chromosomes are aligned in center
12. Final stage of mitosis
13A. Short hairlike structures for movement
13D. Three bases on mRNA
14. Three bases on tRNA
15. Movement of particles from higher to lower concentration
16. Contains RNA within the nucleus
17A. Gel-like fluid within a cell
17D. Response to hypertonic solutions
18. Contains digestive enzymes within the cell
19. Nuclear division in somatic cells
20. Apparatus that "packages" secretory material
21. Base that pairs with guanine

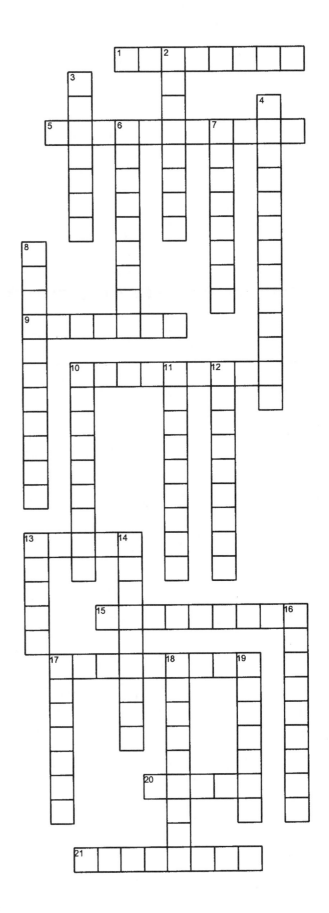

4

Tissues and Membranes

KEY TERMS

Chondrocyte
Collagenous fibers
Elastic fibers
Fibroblast
Histology
Macrophage
Mast cell
Neuroglia
Neuron
Osteocyte
Tissue

BUILDING VOCABULARY

a-
aden-
adip-
ambi-
auscult-
-blast
carcin-
chrondr-
cohes-
erythr-
fibro-
glia-
hist-
inocul-
leuk-
macro-
malign-
multi-
neur-
-oma
os-

pre-
pseudo-
squam-
strat-
stric-
thromb-
tox-
vacu-
vas-

CLINICAL TERMS

Adhesion
Biopsy
Carcinoma
Histology
Lipoma
Marfan's syndrome
Myoma
Papilloma
Pathology
Sarcoma
Scurvy
Systemic lupus erythematosus

CLINICAL ABBREVIATIONS

ac
ASA
D5W
ET
IM
IV
mo
NS
pc

CLINICAL ABBREVIATIONS *(cont'd)*

PO	qid
PR	tiw
qd	yo

OUTLINE/OBJECTIVES

Body Tissues

- List the four main types of tissues found in the body.
  - A tissue is a group of similar cells collected together by an intercellular matrix. Histology is the study of tissues. There are four main types of tissues in the body: epithelial, connective, muscle, and nerve tissue.
- Describe the various types of epithelial tissues in terms of structure, location, functions.
  - Epithelial tissues consist of tightly packed cells with little intercellular matrix, have one free surface, are avascular, and reproduce readily. They cover the body, line body cavities, and cover organs within body cavities. The cells may be squamous, cuboidal, or columnar in shape, and may be arranged in single or multiple layers.
  - Simple squamous epithelium consists of a single layer of flat cells; because it is so thin, it is found in alveoli of lungs and glomerulus of kidneys where it is well suited for diffusion and filtration.
  - Simple cuboidal epithelium consists of a single layer of cells shaped like a cube; it is found in the kidney tubules where it functions in absorption and in glandular tissue where it functions in secretion.
  - Simple columnar epithelium consists of a single layer of cells that are taller than they are wide; it lines the stomach and intestines where it functions in secretion and absorption; microvilli and goblet cells are frequently found in this tissue.
  - Pseudostratified columnar epithelium appears to be stratified but is not; all cells are attached to the basement membrane, but not all reach the surface; cilia and goblet cells are often associated with this tissue; it lines portions of the respiratory tract and some of the tubes of the reproductive tract.
  - Stratified squamous epithelium consists of several layers of cells, and the ones at the surface are flat, squamous cells; protection is the primary function because it is thicker than other epithelia; it forms the outer layer of the skin and the linings of the mouth, anus, and vagina.
  - Transitional epithelium has several layers but can be stretched in response to tension; it is found in the lining of the urinary bladder.
- Describe the classification of glandular epithelium according to structure and method of secretion; give an example of each type.
  - Exocrine glands secrete their product onto a free surface through a duct; endocrine glands are ductless glands and secrete their products into the blood.
  - Goblet cells are unicellular exocrine glands; other exocrine glands are multicellular.
  - The ducts of simple glands have no branches; compound glands have branched ducts; tubular glands have a constant diameter; acinar glands have a saccular distal end.
  - Merocrine glands lose no cytoplasm with their secretion; include salivary glands, pancreatic glands, and most sweat glands.
  - Apocrine glands lose a portion of the cell with the secretory product; include certain sweat glands and mammary glands.
  - In holocrine glands, the entire cell is discharged with the secretory product; includes sebaceous (oil) glands.
- Describe the general characteristics of connective tissues.

— Connective tissue has an abundance of intercellular matrix with relatively few cells.
— Strong and flexible collagenous fibers and yellow elastic fibers are frequently found in the matrix.
- Name three types of connective tissue cells and state the function of each one.
  — Fibroblasts produce the fibers found in connective tissue.
  — Macrophages are phagocytic connective tissue cells that clean up cellular debris and foreign particles.
  — Mast cells contain heparin, an anticoagulant, and histamine, a substance that promotes inflammation.
- Describe the features and location of the various types of connective tissue.
  — Loose connective tissue is characterized by a loose network of collagenous and elastic fibers and a variety of connective tissue cells; the predominant cell is the fibroblast; it fills spaces in the body and binds structures together.
  — Adipose tissue is commonly called fat; it forms a protective cushion around certain organs, provides insulation, and is an efficient energy storage material.
  — Dense fibrous connective tissue is characterized by densely packed collagenous fibers in the matrix; it has a poor vascular supply; forms tendons and ligaments.
  — Cartilage has a matrix that contains the protein chondrin and cells called chondrocytes that are located in spaces called lacunae; it is typically surrounded by a fibrous connective tissue membrane called perichondrium; blood vessels do not penetrate cartilage so cellular reproduction and healing occur slowly; most common type is hyaline cartilage, found at the ends of long bones, trachea, costal cartilages, and fetal skeleton; fibrocartilage has an abundance of collagenous fibers in the matrix and is found in the intervertebral disks; elastic cartilage has an abundance of elastic fibers in the matrix and is found in the framework of the external ear.
  — Bone, or osseous tissue, is a rigid connective tissue with mineral salts in the matrix to give strength and hardness; its structural unit is the osteon, or haversian system. The cells found in bone are osteocytes.
  — Blood is a connective tissue that has a liquid matrix called plasma; its cells are the erythrocytes, which transport oxygen; leukocytes, which fight disease; and thrombocytes, which function in blood clotting.
- Distinguish between skeletal muscle, smooth muscle, and cardiac muscle in terms of structure, location, and control.
  — Actin and myosin are the contractile proteins in muscle tissue.
  — Skeletal muscle fibers are cylindrical, multinucleated, striated, and under voluntary control; skeletal muscles are attached to the skeleton.
  — Smooth muscle cells are spindle-shaped, have a single, centrally located nucleus, lack striations, and are involuntary. Smooth muscle is found in the walls of blood vessels and internal organs.
  — Cardiac muscle cells have branching fibers, one nucleus per cell, striations, intercalated disks, and are involuntary. Cardiac muscle is in the wall of the heart.
- Name two categories of cells in nerve tissue and state their general functions.
  — Neurons and neuroglia are the cells found in nerve tissue.
  — Neurons are the conducting cells of nerve tissue; they have a cell body with efferent processes called axons and afferent processes called dendrites.
  — Neuroglia are the supporting cells of nerve tissue; they do not conduct impulses.

Inflammation and Tissue Repair

- Describe the four manifestations of inflammation and how they develop.
  — The four manifestations of inflammation are redness, swelling, heat, and pain.
  — Blood vessel dilation increases blood flow to the area which causes the redness and heat.

— Increased vascular permeability results in an accumulation of fluid in the tissue spaces, which accounts for the swelling. The swelling puts pressure on the nerves to cause pain.

• Differentiate between regeneration and fibrosis by describing each process.
— Regeneration is the replacement of destroyed tissue by cells that are identical to the original tissue cells.
— Fibrosis is the replacement of destroyed tissue by formation of fibrous connective tissue (scar tissue).
— Most tissue repair is a combination of regeneration and fibrosis.

Body Membranes

• Describe four types of membranes and specify the location and function of each.
— Mucous and serous membranes are epithelial membranes formed from epithelial tissue and the connective tissue to which it is attached. Synovial membranes and the meninges are connective tissue membranes, which contain only connective tissue.
— Mucous membranes are epithelial membranes that line body cavities that open to the outside, such as the mouth, stomach, intestines, urinary bladder, and respiratory tract; they secrete mucus for protection and lubrication.
— Serous membranes are epithelial membranes that line body cavities that do not open to the outside and also cover the organs within these cavities. Serous membranes always consist of two layers, the visceral layer around organs and the parietal layer, which lines cavities. Serous fluid is secreted between the two layers. Pleura is the serous membrane around the lungs, pericardium is around the heart, and peritoneum is in the abdomen.
— Synovial membranes are connective tissue membranes that line joint cavities and secrete a synovial fluid into the joint cavity for lubrication.
— Meninges are connective tissue membranes around the brain and spinal cord. Dura mater is the outer layer of the meninges, arachnoid is the middle layer, and pia mater is the innermost layer.

LEARNING EXERCISES

Body Tissues

1. Write a sentence that defines the term "tissue."

2. The study of tissues is called _____.

3. List the four types of tissues found in the body.

   (a)

   (b)

   (c)

   (d)

4. Complete the description of epithelial tissue by writing the correct words in the blanks.

Epithelial tissues consist of _____ cells with _____ intercellular matrix. They have _____ surface, have no _____ supply, and _____ quickly. These tissues _____ the body, _____ body cavities, and _____ the organs within the body cavities. The cells may be _____, _____, or _____ in shape.

5. Match the following illustrations of epithelial tissues with the correct tissue type and location. Select your answers from the list provided for you.

Type of Epithelium	**Locations**
Simple squamous	Digestive tract
Simple cuboidal	Respiratory passages
Simple columnar with cilia	Urinary bladder
Pseudostratified ciliated columnar	Skin
Stratified squamous	Alveoli of lungs
Transitional	Kidneys

Type _____

Location _____

Type _____

Location _____

Type _____

Location _____

6. Write "endocrine" before each phrase that refers to an endocrine gland and write "exocrine" before each phrase that refers to an exocrine gland.

_____ Ductless gland

_____ Goblet cells

_____ Secrete product onto a surface

_____ Have ducts

_____ Secrete product into blood

7. Match each of the following phrases with the term it best describes. There is one answer for each phrase.

_____ Ducts do not have branches   A. compound

_____ Glandular portion is round   B. simple

_____ Entire cell is discharged with secretion   C. tubular

_____ No cytoplasm is lost with secretion   D. acinar

_____ Portion of cell is lost with secretion   E. merocrine

                                   F. apocrine

                                   G. holocrine

8. Write the terms that match the following phrases about connective tissue.

_____ Fibers that are strong and flexible

_____ Connective tissue cells that are phagocytic

_____ Type that anchors skin to underlying tissues

_____ Type that contains fat

_____ Type that is found in tendons and ligaments

_____ Covering around cartilage

_____ Type of cartilage in intervertebral discs

_____ Most rigid connective tissue

_____ Structural unit of bone

_____ Bone cells

_____ Connective tissue with liquid matrix

_____ Another name for red blood cells

9. Answer the following questions about the accompanying diagram.

   What type of connective tissue is illustrated in this diagram?

   What type of fiber is represented by letter A?

   What type of fiber is represented by letter B?

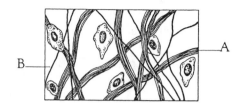

10. Answer the following questions about the accompanying diagram.

    What type of connective tissue is illustrated in this diagram?

    What type of protein is found in the intercellular matrix A?

    What is the name of the cell represented by letter B?

    What is the space represented by letter C?

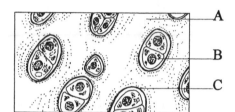

11. Answer the following questions about the accompanying diagram.

    What type of connective tissue is illustrated in this diagram?

    What term is used for the concentric rings of matrix represented by letter A?

    What is the central structure represented by letter B?

    What term is used for the tiny hairlike structures represented by letter C?

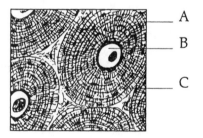

12. Answer the following questions about the accompanying diagram.

    What type of muscle tissue is illustrated in this diagram?

    What term is used for the cell membrane represented by letter A?

    What two types of contractile proteins are found in this tissue?

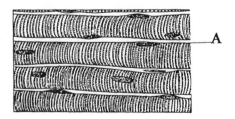

13. Answer the following questions about the accompanying diagram.

    What type of muscle tissue is illustrated in this diagram?

    Give two locations for this type of muscle tissue.

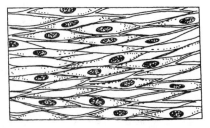

14. Answer the following questions about the accompanying diagram.

    What type of muscle tissue is illustrated in this diagram?

    What is the term for the dark band represented by letter B?

    Where is this type of muscle located?

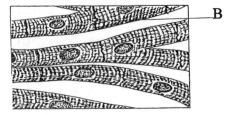

15. Write the terms that match the following phrases about nervous tissue.

    _____ Cells that transmit impulses

    _____ Take impulses to cell body

    _____ Take impulses away from cell body

    _____ Supporting cells of nerve tissue

Inflammation and Tissue Repair

1. Which characteristics of inflammation result from

   a. blood vessel dilation

   b. increased vascular permeability

2. Indicate whether each of the following phrases pertains to regeneration (R) or fibrosis (F).

   _____ Scar tissue

   _____ Surface abrasions

   _____ Cells identical to original cells

   _____ Granulation tissue

   _____ Occurs only in tissues capable of mitosis

   _____ Occurs in skeletal muscle

   _____ Proliferation of collagen fibers

Body Membranes

1. Write the terms that match the following phrases about body membranes.

_____ Membranes composed only of connective tissue

_____ Line cavities that open to the outside

_____ Type of membrane lining digestive tract

_____ Membranes with two layers

_____ Layer that lines a cavity wall

_____ Layer that covers organs within a cavity

_____ Serous membrane associated with the lungs

_____ Serous membrane associated with the heart

_____ Serous membrane of abdominopelvic cavity

_____ Connective tissue membrane of movable joints

_____ Connective tissue membranes around the brain

_____ Tough, outermost layer of meninges

_____ Middle layer of the meninges

_____ Innermost layer of the meninges

REVIEW QUESTIONS

1. What constitutes a tissue?
2. What is the term given to the microscopic study of tissues?
3. Name the four main types of tissues found in the body.
4. List five functions of epithelial tissues and tell where these tissues are located.
5. Which item in each of the following pairs of items refers to epithelial tissue?
    (a) relatively large amount of matrix; relatively small amount of matrix
    (b) poor mitotic capabilities; readily mitotic
    (c) abundant blood supply; has no blood vessels
    (d) closely packed cells; scattered cells
    (e) always surrounded by other tissues; always has a free surface
6. What is the difference between simple epithelium and stratified epithelium?
7. Describe the appearance of each of the following:
    (a) simple squamous epithelium
    (b) simple columnar epithelium
    (c) pseudostratified columnar epithelium
    (d) stratified squamous epithelium
8. Indicate where each of the following is found:
    (a) simple cuboidal epithelium
    (b) simple columnar epithelium

(c) transitional epithelium

(d) stratified squamous epithelium

9. What is the difference between exocrine and endocrine glands?

10. What type of gland are goblet cells?

11. What is the difference in shape between tubular glands and alveolar glands?

12. What is the difference among merocrine, apocrine, and holocrine glands?

13. Compare the structural features of connective tissue with the structural features of epithelial tissue.

14. Describe the characteristics of collagenous fibers and elastic fibers.

15. What is the function of each of the following cells: fibroblast, macrophage, mast cell?

16. What is another name for loose connective tissue? Where is it found?

17. How does dense fibrous connective tissue differ from loose connective tissue? Where is dense fibrous connective tissue located?

18. Use the following terms in a description of cartilage: chondrin, chondrocytes, lacunae, perichondrium.

19. What is the difference in structure between hyaline cartilage, fibrocartilage, and elastic cartilage? Where is each type located?

20. Use the following terms in a description of the structure of osseous tissue: osteon, haversian canal, lamellae, osteocytes, lacunae, canaliculi.

21. What is the term for each of the following: red blood cells, white blood cells, platelets, intercellular matrix of blood?

22. What are actin and myosin?

23. Indicate whether each of the following pertains to skeletal muscle, smooth muscle, or cardiac muscle.
    (a) multinucleated
    (b) intercalated disks
    (c) spindle-shaped cells
    (d) cross-striations
    (e) located in the wall of internal organs
    (f) under voluntary control

24. What is the difference between neurons and neuroglia?

25. Use the terms axon, dendrite, and cell body in a description of the neuron.

26. What are the characteristics and benefits of inflammation?

27. What are the two types of tissue repair and which one produces scar tissue?

28. What is the difference in structure between epithelial membranes and connective tissue membranes?

29. Where are mucous membranes located?

30. Where are serous membranes located?

31. Describe the specific location for each of the following:
    (a) parietal pleura
    (b) visceral pericardium
    (c) parietal peritoneum

32. What type of membrane is described by each of the following?
    (a) lines joint cavities
    (b) surrounds the brain and spinal cord
    (c) one layer is the dura mater

CHAPTER QUIZ

1. Match each description or component with the correct tissue type.

    _____ Closely packed cells   A. epithelium

    _____ Macrophages and fibroblasts   B. connective

    _____ Tendons and ligaments   C. muscle

    _____ Simple and stratified   D. nerve

    _____ Axons and dendrites

    _____ Chondrocytes and osteocytes

    _____ Specialized for contraction

    _____ Blood and bones

    _____ Has a free surface

    _____ Actin and myosin

2. Match each of the following locations with the correct tissue type. Some responses may be used more than once, others may not be used at all.

    _____ Outer layer of skin   A. adipose

    _____ Kidney tubules   B. dense fibrous connective tissue

    _____ Costal cartilage   C. elastic cartilage

    _____ Attaches skin to muscles   D. fibrocartilage

    _____ Lining of the stomach   E. hyaline cartilage

    _____ Most of the fetal skeleton   F. loose connective tissue

    _____ Alveoli of the lungs, for diffusion G. simple columnar epithelium

    _____ Tendons   H. simple cuboidal epithelium

    _____ Lining of the urinary bladder   I. simple squamous epithelium

    _____ Intervertebral disks   J. smooth muscle

                                             K. stratified squamous epithelium

                                             L. transitional epithelium

3. Ductless glands, which secrete their product directly into the blood, are called
    _____ glands.

4. Goblet cells are an example of (a) endocrine glands, (b) merocrine glands, (c) apocrine glands, (d) unicellular glands.

5. Ligaments have an abundance of (a) blood vessels, (b) mast cells, (c) elastic fibers, (d) adipose cells, (e) collagenous fibers.

6. Which of the following is found in both osseous tissue and cartilage? (a) canaliculi, (b) lamellae, (c) lacunae, (d) haversian canals.

7. Another name for a platelet is _____.

8. Involuntary control and cross-striations are characteristic of (a) skeletal muscle, (b) smooth muscle, (c) visceral muscle, (d) cardiac muscle.

9. The processes on neurons that carry impulses away from the cell body are called

   _____.

10. Membranes that line body cavities that open to the exterior are (a) mucous membranes, (b) synovial membranes, (c) serous membranes, (d) meninges.

USING CLINICAL KNOWLEDGE

1. Match the definitions on the left with the correct term from the column on the right by placing the corresponding letter in the space before the definition. Not all terms will be used.

_____	Study that involves the absorption and distribution of a drug	A. Adhesion
_____	Tumor derived from fat cells	B. Biopsy
_____	Abnormal joining of tissues by scar tissue	C. Carcinoma
_____	Cells that release histamine in allergic reactions	D. Lipoma
_____	Removal and microscopic examination of tissues	E. Macrophage
_____	Study of the structural and functional changes in tissues caused by disease	F. Mast cell
		G. Pathology
_____	Malignant growth derived from connective tissue cells	H. Pharmacodynamics
		I. Pharmacokinetics
_____	Malignant growth derived from epithelial cells	J. Sarcoma

2. Write the meaning of the following abbreviations.

    _____ D5W

    _____ NS

    _____ IM

    _____ tiw

    _____ ASA

3. Spelling is important in scientific and medical applications because only one or two incorrect letters may change the meaning. Two of the following words from this chapter are misspelled. Place a check mark (√) in the space before the word if it is spelled correctly. Write the correct spelling in the space if it is spelled incorrectly.

    _____ skurvy

    _____ macrophage

    _____ condrocyte

    _____ neuroglia

    _____ papilloma

4. For each of the following words, underline the root and write the meaning of the root on the line preceding the word.

    _____ vacuous

    _____ auscultation

_____ cohesive

_____ stricture

_____ adipose

_____ stratified

_____ inoculation

5. Write the meaning of the underlined portion of the following words on the line preceding each word.

_____ <u>macro</u>phage

_____ <u>pseudo</u>stratified

_____ <u>multi</u>nuclear

_____ osteo<u>blast</u>

_____ carcin<u>oma</u>

_____ <u>aden</u>oma

_____ <u>neuro</u>glia

_____ neuro<u>glia</u>

_____ <u>erythro</u>cyte

_____ <u>squam</u>ous

FUN AND GAMES

Each of the answers in this puzzle is a term from this chapter on tissues and membranes. Fill in the answers to the clues by using syllables from the list that is provided. The number of syllables in each word is indicated by the number in parentheses after the clue. The number of letters in each word is indicated by the number of spaces provided. All syllables in the list are to be used and no syllable is used more than once unless it is duplicated in the list.

A	CYTE	LAGE	O	RON
A	E	LAR	PHAGE	RYTH
AD	EP	LI	PLEU	SQUA
AL	FI	MAC	POSE	SYN
AL	GES	MEN	RA	TA
BRO	GLI	MOUS	RE	THE
CAR	HIS	MINE	RO	TI
CER	I	NEU	RO	UM
CHOND	I	NEU	RO	VI
CYTE	IN	O	RO	VIS

Tissue filled with fat (3)   __ __ __ __ __ __ __

Conducts impulses (2)   __ __ __ __ __ __

A serous membrane (2)   __ __ __ __ __ __

Cartilage cell (3)   __ __ __ __ __ __ __ __ __ __

Tissue that forms coverings (5)   __ __ __ __ __ __ __ __ __ __

Membranes around the brain (3)   __ __ __ __ __ __ __ __

Large phagocytic cell (3)   __ __ __ __ __ __ __ __ __

Substance in mast cells (3)   __ __ __ __ __ __ __ __

Red blood cell (4)   __ __ __ __ __ __ __ __ __ __ __

Loose connective tissue (4)   __ __ __ __ __ __ __

Smooth muscle (3)   __ __ __ __ __ __ __

Membrane in movable joints (4)   __ __ __ __ __ __ __ __ __

Flat epithelial cells (2)   __ __ __ __ __ __ __

Tissue in intervertebral disks (5)   __ __ __ __ __ __ __ __ __ __ __ __

Nerve glue (4)   __ __ __ __ __ __ __ __ __ __

5

Integumentary System

KEY TERMS

Arrector pili
Ceruminous gland
Dermis
Epidermis
Keratinization
Melanin
Sebaceous gland
Subcutaneous layer
Sudoriferous gland

BUILDING VOCABULARY

albin-
cer-
-cidal
cry-
cutane-
cyan-
derm-
-ectomy
erythem-
hidr-
ichthy-
kerat-
-lucid-
melan-
mes-
myc-
necr-
onych-
pachy-
pedicul-
pil-
-plasty
rhytid-
seb-
sud-
trich-
ungu-
xer-

CLINICAL TERMS

Alopecia
Basal cell carcinoma
Cellulitis
Dermatitis
Eczema
Eschar
Hives
Impetigo
Malignant melanoma
Nevus
Pruritus
Urticaria
Wart
Xeroderma pigmentosum

CLINICAL ABBREVIATIONS

ADR
ADT
BFP
bx
EAHF
HSV
I&D
M&F
subq, sub-Q
SCC
SG
ung
UV
XP

OUTLINE/OBJECTIVES

Structure of the Skin

- Describe the structure of the two layers of the skin.
  - The integumentary system includes the skin with its glands, hair, and nails. The skin has an outer epidermis and an inner dermis. These are anchored to underlying tissues by the hypodermis or subcutaneous tissue.
  - The epidermis is stratified squamous epithelium. In thick skin, it has five distinct regions.
  - The bottom layer of the epidermis is the stratum basale. It is closest to the blood supply, is actively mitotic, and contains melanocytes.
  - The other layers are the stratum spinosum, stratum granulosum, stratum lucidum (present only in thick skin), and stratum corneum.
  - The outermost layer, the stratum corneum, is continually sloughed off and replaced by cells from deeper layers.
  - The dermis, also called stratum corium, is composed of connective tissue with blood vessels, nerves, and accessory structures embedded in it. It consists of two layers, the upper papillary layer and the deeper reticular layer.
- Name the supporting layer of the skin and describe its structure.
  - The hypodermis, also called subcutaneous tissue, anchors the skin to the underlying muscles. The hypodermis is connective tissue with an abundance of adipose, which acts as a cushion and a heat insulator, and can be used as an energy source.

Skin Color

- Discuss three factors that influence skin color.
  - Basic skin color is due to the amount of melanin produced by the melanocytes in the stratum basale.
  - Carotene, a yellow pigment, gives a yellow tint to the skin.
  - Blood in the dermal blood vessels gives a pink color to the skin.

Epidermal Derivatives

- Describe the structure of hair and nails and their relationship to the skin.
  - The central core of hair is the medulla, which is surrounded by the cortex and the cuticle. Hair is divided into the visible shaft and the root, which is embedded in the skin and surrounded by the follicle. The distal end of the hair follicle expands to form a bulb around a central papilla.
  - Stratum basale cells in the bulb undergo mitosis to form hair, which increases the length of the hair. Hair color is determined by melanocytes in the stratum basale.
  - Arrector pili muscle contracts in response to cold and fear to make the hair "stand on end."
  - Nails are thin plates of keratinized stratum corneum. Each nail has a free edge, nail body, and a nail root. Other structures associated with the nail are the nail bed, nail matrix, eponychium, and lunula.
  - Nails are derived from the stratum basale in the nail bed.
- Discuss the characteristics and functions of the various glands associated with the skin.
  - Sebaceous glands are oil glands and are associated with hair follicles. These glands secrete sebum, which helps keep hair and skin soft and pliable and helps prevent water loss.
  - Sweat glands are called sudoriferous glands. Merocrine sweat glands open to the surface of the skin through sweat pores and secrete perspiration in response to nerve stimulation and in response to heat.

— Apocrine sweat glands are larger than merocrine glands and their distribution is limited to the axillae and external genitalia where they open into hair follicles. These glands become active at puberty and are stimulated in response to pain, emotional stress, and sexual arousal.

— Ceruminous glands are modified sweat glands found only in the external auditory canal where they secrete cerumen, or earwax.

Functions of the Skin

• Discuss four functions of the integumentary system.
  — Protection: The skin protects against water loss, invading organisms, ultraviolet light, and other injuries.
  — Sensory reception: Sense receptors in the skin detect information about the environment and also serve as a means of communication between individuals.
  — Regulation of body temperature: Constriction and dilation of blood vessels affect the amount of heat that escapes from the skin into the surrounding air. Sweat glands are stimulated in response to heat and are inactive in cold temperatures. Adipose in the subcutaneous tissue helps insulate the body.
  — Synthesis of vitamin D: Precursors for vitamin D are found in the skin. When the skin is exposed to ultraviolet light, these precursors are converted into active vitamin D.

Burns

• Discuss the characteristics of first, second, and third degree burns.
  — First degree burns are superficial, involve only the epidermis, are red and painful, and heal by regeneration.
  — Second degree burns are partial thickness burns, involve a portion of the dermis, form blisters, are painful, and may produce scarring.
  — Third degree burns are full thickness burns, which extend into the subcutaneous tissue or below. They are white or charred, cause no pain, present problems with fluid loss and infection, and produce severe scarring.
• Explain the rule of nines.
  — The rule of nines may be used to estimate the amount of body surface area that is burned.
  — Each body region constitutes a percentage of the total that is a multiple of nine.
  — Head and neck total 9%, each upper extremity is 9%, each lower limb is 18%, the entire trunk is 36%, and the perineum is 1%.

LEARNING EXERCISES

Structure of the Skin

1. The integumentary system includes _____, _____, _____, and _____.

2. Write the name of the layer or structure that corresponds to each of the descriptions. Select your answers from the following choices.

Dermis   Stratum basale   Stratum granulosum
Epidermis   Stratum corneum   Stratum lucidum
Hypodermis   Stratum germinativum   Stratum spinosum

_____ Referred to as the subcutaneous layer

_____ Specific layer that contains melanocytes

_____ Epidermal layer next to the dermis

_____ Consists of stratum basale and stratum spinosum

_____ Consists of a papillary layer and a reticular layer

_____ Layer immediately above the stratum basale

_____ Referred to as superficial fascia

_____ Found only in thick skin

_____ Keratinization begins in this layer

_____ Consists of dead, completely keratinized cells

_____ Layer in which hair, nails, and glands are embedded

_____ Contains receptors for temperature and touch

_____ Contains adipose tissue

_____ Actively mitotic layer

_____ Has collagen fibers that give strength to the skin

3. Identify the layers and structures of the skin in the following diagram by placing the correct letter in the space provided by the listed labels. Then select different colors for each structure and use them to color the coding circles and the corresponding structures in the illustration.

_____ Arrector pili muscle ○

_____ Blood vessel ○

_____ Epidermis ○

_____ Hair bulb ○

_____ Sebaceous gland ○

_____ Stratum basale ○

_____ Stratum corneum ○

_____ Sweat gland ○

Skin Color

1. What is the name of the dark pigment that is primarily responsible for skin color?

2. What is the name of the yellow pigment found in the skin?

3. What accounts for the pink color of the skin?

4. Explain why a "tan" is temporary.

Epidermal Derivatives

1. Write the terms that fit the following descriptive phrases about epidermal derivatives.

_____ Tubular sheath surrounding the hair root

_____ Smooth muscle associated with hair

_____ Epidermal layer that produces hair and nails

_____ Central core of a hair

_____ Crescent-shaped area over the nail matrix

_____ Type of gland generally associated with hair

_____ Glands that produce earwax

_____ Sweat glands that function in temperature regulation

_____ Another name for sweat glands

_____ Enlarged region of hair follicle embedded in dermis

_____ Another name for nail cuticle

_____ Large sweat glands in the axilla

Functions of the Skin

1. Four types of functions of the integument are:

    (a)

    (b)

    (c)

    (d)

2. The protein that is a waterproofing agent in the skin is _____.

3. Bacterial growth on the skin is inhibited by _____.

4. Tissues under the skin are protected from ultraviolet light by _____.

5. Sense receptors for heat, cold, pain, touch, and pressure are located in the _____ of the skin.

6. Describe two mechanisms by which the skin functions in temperature regulation.

    (a) blood vessels

    (b) sweat glands

7. How does the skin function in the synthesis of vitamin D?

Burns

1. Indicate whether each of the following phrases pertains to first degree (1), second degree (2), or third degree (3) burns. If the phrase pertains to more than one type, indicate this by using all the correct numbers.

   _____   requires skin grafts

   _____   stratum basale damaged

   _____   heals by regeneration

   _____   becomes red

   _____   involves subcutaneous tissue

   _____   painful

   _____   blisters

   _____   superficial

   _____   may produce scarring

   _____   involves the dermis

   _____   severe scarring

   _____   nerve endings destroyed

2. Jack B. Nimble suffered third degree burns over his anterior trunk and the anterior surface of both arms.

   a. What percentage of his total body surface area had third degree burns?

   b. What are the two most important medical challenges presented by this burn?

REVIEW QUESTIONS

1. What structures make up the integumentary system?
2. What are the epidermis, dermis, and hypodermis?
3. Name the five layers of the epidermis of thick skin and describe the appearance of each layer.
4. What are the features of the two layers of the dermis?
5. Describe two functions of the hypodermis.
6. Discuss two ways in which the integument helps to regulate body temperature.
7. What is the primary factor that determines skin color? Name two additional factors.
8. From what tissue are hair and fingernails derived?

9. Use the following terms in a description of the structure of hair: shaft, root, medulla, cortex, cuticle, hair follicle, hair bulb, papilla, and arrector pili muscle.

10. Use the following terms in a description of the structure of nails: free edge, nail body, nail root, eponychium, nail bed, nail matrix, and lunula.

11. Where are sebaceous glands located? What is their secretory product? What is their function?

12. What is the difference between merocrine and apocrine sudoriferous glands? Where are they located?

13. What are ceruminous glands and where are they located?

14. List four functions of the skin.

15. What are the most serious medical challenges from severe burns?

16. Which two types of burns are painful?

17. Name the skin layers that are damaged in first, second, and third degree burns.

CHAPTER QUIZ

1. Match each of the following descriptions with the correct layer of the skin.

    _____ Outermost layer   A. dermis

    _____ Responsible for fingerprints   B. epidermis

    _____ Has five distinct layers in thick skin   C. hypodermis

    _____ Contains adipose

    _____ Has cells responsible for skin color

    _____ Stratified squamous epithelium

    _____ Hair and nails are derived from this layer

    _____ Has sense receptors and hair embedded in it

2. The central core of hair is the
    (a) medulla
    (b) cortex
    (c) shaft
    (d) follicle
    (e) cuticle

3. Which of the following is *not* associated with hair?
    (a) arrector pili
    (b) sebaceous glands
    (c) stratum basale
    (d) apocrine sweat glands
    (e) merocrine sweat glands

4. Which one of the following statements is *not* true about functions of the skin?
    (a) exposure to ultraviolet light usually increases the activity of melanocytes
    (b) secretions of sweat glands help protect against fluid loss
    (c) when body temperatures increase, the dermal capillaries dilate
    (d) vitamin D is produced in the skin in response to ultraviolet light

5. (True or False) All people have approximately the same number of melanocytes.

6. Which of the following does not describe a third degree burn?
   (a) hypodermis is involved
   (b) blisters form
   (c) results in scarring
   (d) full-thickness burn

USING CLINICAL KNOWLEDGE

1. Match the definitions on the left with the correct term from the column on the right by placing the corresponding letter in the space before the definition. Not all terms will be used.

_____	Deepest layer of skin damaged in a second degree burn	A.	Alopecia
_____	Baldness	B.	Dermatitis
_____	Sunscreen preparation	C.	Dermis
_____	A slough produced by a burn or gangrene	D.	Epidermis
_____	Severe itching	E.	Eschar
_____	A mole	F.	Nevus
_____	Inflammation of the skin	G.	Prophylactic agent
_____	Hives	H.	Pruritus
		I.	Therapeutic agent
		J.	Urticaria

2. Write the meaning of the following abbreviations.

_____ UV

_____ EAHF

_____ ung

_____ HSV

_____ I&D

3. Spelling is important in scientific and medical applications because only one or two incorrect letters may change the meaning. Two of the following words from this chapter are misspelled. Place a check mark (√) in the space before the word if it is spelled correctly. Write the correct spelling in the space if it is spelled incorrectly.

_____ eczema

_____ impetigo

_____ carotinization

_____ sebacious

_____ subcutaneous

4. Write the meaning of the underlined portion of each word on the line preceding the word.

_____ <u>cer</u>uminous

_____ <u>sud</u>oriferous

_____ <u>ichthy</u>osis

_____	hyp<u>onych</u>ium
_____	gastr<u>ectomy</u>
_____	dermato<u>plasty</u>
_____	<u>xer</u>oderma
_____	bacteri<u>cidal</u>
_____	<u>cyan</u>osis
_____	<u>pediculo</u>sis

5. Separate each of the following words into its component parts, give the meaning of each part, then write the meaning of the entire word.

Hidradenitis:

_____

_____

Mycodermatitis:

_____

_____

_____

FUN AND GAMES

Complete this crossword puzzle by filling in the answers to the clues. Clues for words from this chapter are highlighted in bold print.

ACROSS
1. **Dermal layer**
7. **Dead skin layer**
12. Honey or bumble
13. Edge
14. Midwest state
15. Ages
17. **Yellow pigment**
19. Hunt
21. Health career, abb.
22. To travel
23. Opposite of down
24. **Skin layer**
28. Border
31. Grad. class
32. Top ones
34. News source
36. Su'mat, Latin abb.
37. Golf clubs
40. Pointed instrument
42. Large
43. Salt
45. **Pigment cell**
46. You and me
47. Tell's target
49. Prefix for within
50. Ruby or emerald
53. Tablecloths
54. Part of Ner. Sys.
56. 33 1/3 record
57. Chicago transport
58. Astatine symbol
59. Nonrigid airship
62. Inten. care units
64. Scat
65. Actinium symbol
67. Lair
68. 24 hours
70. **Below the skin**
75. Oper. rm.
76. Hoover or Cooley
78. Private teacher
79. See 56 across
80. **Subcutaneous**
83. Denoting presence
84. Repast
86. Illinium symbol
87. Past part. of lie
89. Second cerv. vert.
90. **Narrow lines or bands**
92. Most sick
94. **Integument**
95. Brit. Ortho. Assoc.
96. Fargo state
97. Univ. of Edinburgh
98. Choose
99. **Clear layer**
101. Prompt, hint
102. Woman, Fr.
104. Call for help
105. One at random
106. **Surrounds muscles and organs**
107. Senescent

DOWN
1. Raise
2. Spooky
3. **Skin**
4. Large vessel or vase
5. Falsehood
6. Before noon
7. Female students
8. Prefix for again
9. Agrees with standard
10. See 49 across
11. 50 states
12. Opposite of AD
14. Med. Examiner
16. Male parent
18. Chances, probability
19. **Epidermal layer**
20. **Epidermal protein**
25. Inspirator capacity
26. **Oil**
27. **Epidermal layer**
29. River in Egypt
30. **Epidermal layer**
33. Suffix denoting condition
35. **Upper dermal layer**
38. Every night, L., abb.
39. Scandium symbol
41. You and I
44. Lic. Prac. Nurse
48. Escape

51. **Upon the skin**
52. Hertz, abb.
55. **Perspiration**
56. **Moon-shaped nail region**
59. Bill of Health, abb.
60. Promissory note
61. Pacific, abb.
63. Head of a company
66. **Pertaining to skin**
68. Capital of Qatar; to laugh
69. Forearm bones
71. **Bottom layer of epidermis**
72. Sound of disapproval
73. Negative
74. Braced
76. Bring to pass
77. **Dark pigment**
81. Corolla of a flower
82. Hip bone
85. Dog native to Greenland
88. Chicago or Rockford state
89. Community college
90. Spheno-occipital junction
91. Small whirlpool
93. Research instrument, abb.
95. Public transport vehicle
100. Calcium symbol
101. Cancer, abbrev.
102. Fatty acid
103. Metric unit

6

Skeletal System

KEY TERMS

Amphiarthrosis
Diaphysis
Diarthrosis
Endochondral ossification
Epiphyseal plate
Epiphysis
Intramembranous ossification
Osterblast
Osteoclast
Osteocyte
Osteon
Synarthrosis

BUILDING VOCABULARY

acetabul-
ankyl-
appendicul-
arthr-
artic-
-blast
burs-
carp-
-clast
corac-
cost-
cribr-
crist-
ethm-
-fic-
ili-
kyph-
myel-
odont-
-oid

oste-,oss-
-poie-
sacr-
sphen-
spondyl-
syn-
-tion

CLINICAL TERMS

Ankylosing spondylitis
Arthritis
Bunion
Carpal tunnel syndrome
Dislocation
Gout
Lyme disease
Osteoarthritis
Osteomalacia
Osteomyelitis
Osteoporosis
Osteosarcoma
Rheumatoid arthritis
Spina bifida
Sprain
Talipes

CLINICAL ABBREVIATIONS

C-1, C-2, etc
CTS
DIPJ
DJD
fx
jt
kj

CLINICAL ABBREVIATIONS *(cont'd)*

lig	SI
NSAID	Sx
OA	T-1, T-2, etc.
RA	Tx
ROM	

OUTLINE/OBJECTIVES

Overview of the Skeletal System

- Discuss five functions of the skeletal system.
  - Bones support the soft organs of the body and support the body against the pull of gravity.
  - Bones protect soft body parts such as the brain, spinal cord, and heart.
  - Bones work with muscles to produce movement.
  - Bones store minerals, especially calcium.
  - Most blood cell formation, hematopoiesis, occurs in red bone marrow.
- Distinguish between compact and spongy bone on the basis of structural features.
  - The microscopic unit of compact bone is the osteon or haversian system. It consists of an osteonic canal, lamellae of matrix, osteocytes in lacunae, and canaliculi. In compact bone, the osteons are packed closely together.
  - Spongy bone is less dense than compact bone and consists of bone trabeculae around irregular cavities that contain red bone marrow. The trabeculae are organized to provide maximum strength to a bone.
- Classify bones according to size and shape and identify the general features of a long bone.
  - Long bones are longer than they are wide; an example is the femur in the thigh.
  - Short bones are roughly cube-shaped; an example is the bones of the wrist.
  - Flat bones have inner and outer tables of compact bone with a diploe of spongy bone in the middle; examples include the bones of the cranium.
  - Irregular bones are primarily spongy bone with a thin layer of compact bone; examples include the vertebrae.
  - Long bones have a diaphysis around a medullary cavity, with an epiphysis at each end. The epiphysis is covered by articular cartilage. Except in the region of the articular cartilage, long bones are covered by periosteum and lined with endosteum. All bones have surface markings that make each one unique.
- Discuss the processes by which bones develop and grow.
  - Bone development is called osteogenesis.
  - Osteoblasts, osteocytes, and osteoclasts are three types of cells involved in bone formation and remodeling.
  - Intramembranous ossification involves the replacement of connective tissue membranes by bone tissue. Flat bones of the skull develop this way.
  - Most bones develop by endochondral ossification. In this process, the bones first form as hyaline cartilage models, which are later replaced by bone.
  - Long bones increase in length at the cartilaginous epiphyseal plate. When the epiphyseal plate completely ossifies, increase in length is no longer possible.
  - Increase in diameter of long bones occurs by appositional growth. Osteoclasts break down old bone next to the medullary cavity at the same time osteoblasts form new bone on the surface.
- Distinguish between the axial and appendicular skeletons, and state the number of bones in each.

— The adult human skeleton has 206 named bones in addition to varying numbers of wormian and sesamoid bones.
— The axial skeleton, with 80 bones, forms the vertical axis of the body. It includes the skull, vertebrae, ribs, and sternum.
— The appendicular skeleton, with 126 bones, includes the appendages and their attachments to the axial skeleton.

Bones of the Axial Skeleton

• Identify the bones of the skull and their important surface markings.
    — The skull includes the bones of the cranium, face, and the auditory ossicles.
    — With the exception of the mandible, the cranial and facial bones are joined by immovable joints called sutures.
    — The eight cranial bones are frontal (1), parietal (2), temporal (2), occipital (1), ethmoid (1), and sphenoid (1). The frontal, ethmoid, and sphenoid bones contain cavities called paranasal sinuses.
    — The 14 bones of the face are maxillae (2), nasal (2), lacrimal (2), zygomatic (2), vomer (1), inferior nasal conchae (2), palatine (2), and mandible (1). Each maxilla contains a large maxillary paranasal sinus.
    — Six auditory ossicles, three in each ear, are located in the temporal bone.
    — The hyoid bone is a U-shaped bone in the neck. It does not articulate with any other bone and functions as a base for the tongue and as an attachment for muscles.
• Identify the general structural features of vertebrae and compare cervical, thoracic, lumbar, sacral, and coccygeal vertebrae; state the number of each type.
    — The vertebral column contains 26 vertebrae that are separated by intervertebral disks.
    — Four curvatures add strength and resiliency to the column. The thoracic and sacral curvatures are concave anteriorly; the cervical and lumbar curvatures are convex anteriorly.
    — All vertebrae have a body or centrum, a vertebral arch, a vertebral foramen, transverse processes, and a spinous process.
    — The seven cervical vertebrae have bifid spinous processes and transverse foramina. The first two cervical vertebrae are unique; the atlas C1, is a ring that holds up the occipital bone; the axis, C2, has a dens or odontoid process.
    — The 12 thoracic vertebrae have facets on the bodies and transverse processes for articulation with the ribs.
    — The five lumbar vertebrae have large heavy bodies to support body weight.
    — The sacrum is formed from five separate bones that fuse together in the adult.
    — The coccyx is the most distal part of the vertebral column. Three to five bones fuse to form the coccyx.
• Identify the structural features of the ribs and sternum.
    — The thoracic cage consists of the thoracic vertebrae, the ribs, and the sternum.
    — The sternum has three parts: the manubrium, the body, and the xiphoid. The jugular notch in the manubrium is an important landmark. The sternal angle is where the manubrium joins the body
    — There are seven pairs of true ribs (vertebrosternal ribs), and five pairs of false ribs. The upper three pairs of false ribs are vertebrochondral, the lower two pairs are vertebral or floating ribs.

Bones of the Appendicular Skeleton

• Identify the features of the pectoral girdle and upper extremity.
    — The pectoral girdle is formed by two clavicles and two scapulas; it supports the upper extremities.

— The upper extremity includes the humerus, radius, ulna, carpus, metacarpus, and phalanges.
— The humerus is the bone in the arm, or brachium; in the forearm, the radius is the lateral bone and the ulna is the medial bone.
— The hand is composed of a wrist, palm, and five fingers. The wrist, or carpus, contains eight small carpal bones; the palm, or metacarpus, contains five metacarpal bones; the 14 bones of the fingers are phalanges.
• Identify the features of the pelvic girdle and lower extremity.
— The pelvic girdle consists of two ossa coxae, or innominate bones, and attaches the lower extremities to the axial skeleton and provides support for the weight of the body.
— Each os coxa is formed by three bones fused together: ilium, ischium, and pubis. The two ossa coxae meet anteriorly at the symphysis pubis.
— The ilium, ischium, and pubis meet in a large cavity, the acetabulum, that provides articulation for the femur.
— The false pelvis (greater pelvis) is the area between the flared portions of the ilium bones; the true pelvis (lesser pelvis) is inferior to the false pelvis and begins at the pelvic brim.
— The bones in the lower extremity are the femur, tibia, fibula, patella, tarsal bones, metatarsals, and phalanges.
— The bone in the thigh is the femur, which articulates in the acetabulum of the os coxa. Distally, the femur articulates with the tibia.
— The medial bone in the leg is the tibia. Proximally it articulates with the femur, distally with the talus. The lateral bone in the leg is the fibula.
— Seven tarsal bones form the ankle. The talus is the tarsal bone that articulates with the tibia. The calcaneus is the heel bone. Five metatarsals form the instep of the foot and there are 14 phalanges in the toes of each foot.
— The patella is a sesamoid bone in the anterior portion of the knee joint.

Fractures and Fracture Repair

• Identify these fractures by description and on diagrams: complete, incomplete, open, closed, transverse, spiral, comminuted, and displaced.
— In a complete fracture, the break extends across the entire section of bone; in an incomplete fracture, there are pieces of the bone partially joined together.
— An open fracture has the bone protruding through the skin and is also called a compound fracture; a closed fracture is a simple fracture where the bone does not extend through the skin.
— The bone is broken at right angles to the long axis of the bone in transverse fractures; in spiral fractures, the bone is broken by twisting.
— If the bone is crushed into small pieces, it is a comminuted fracture; if the pieces of bone are not in correct alignment, it is a displaced fracture.
• Describe the process of fracture repair by using the terms fracture hematoma, procallus, fibrocartilaginous callus, bony callus, and remodeling.
— Blood vessels are torn when a bone breaks and the blood from these vessels clots to form a fracture hematoma.
— New capillaries start to grow into the fracture hematoma and organize it into a procallus.
— Fibroblasts from neighboring healthy tissue migrate to the fracture area and produce collagen fibers within the procallus; chondroblasts produce fibrocartilage that transforms the procallus into a fibrocartilaginous callus.
— Osteoblasts infiltrate the fibrocartilaginous callus and produce trabeculae of spongy bone to form a bony callus.
— Remodeling is the final step. In this process osteoblasts and osteoclasts remodel the bony callus into the original configuration of compact bone and spongy bone.

Articulations

- Compare the structure and function of three types of joints.
  - Synarthroses are immovable joints where the bones are held together by short fibers; sutures are synarthrotic joints.
  - Slightly movable joints are amphiarthroses. In this type of joint, the bones are connected by hyaline cartilage or fibrocartilage. The symphysis pubis and intervertebral disks are examples of amphiarthrotic joints.
  - Joints that are freely movable are diarthroses. In this type of joint, the bones are held together by a fibrous joint capsule that is lined with synovial membrane. These joints are sometimes called synovial joints. There are six types of synovial joints, based on the shape of the opposing bones and the type of motion: gliding, condyloid, hinge, saddle, pivot, and ball-and-socket.

LEARNING EXERCISES

Overview of the Skeletal System

1. List five functions of the skeletal system.

   (a)

   (b)

   (c)

   (d)

   (e)

2. Place an S before each phrase that pertains to spongy bone and a C before each phrase that pertains to compact bone.

   _____ Closely packed osteons

   _____ Contains red bone marrow

   _____ Trabeculae

   _____ Canaliculi radiate from lacunae to osteonic canal

   _____ Contains irregular spaces

3. Place an L before each phrase that pertains to long bones, an S before each phrase that pertains to short bones, and an F before each phrase that pertains to flat bones.

   _____ Has a diploe of spongy bone

   _____ Vertical dimension longer than the horizontal dimension

   _____ Roughly cube-shaped

   _____ Primarily spongy bone covered with a thin layer of compact bone

   _____ Bones in the wrist and ankle

   _____ Bones in the thigh and arm

   _____ Spongy bone between two layers of compact bone

4. Write the terms that fit the following descriptive phrases about the features of long bone.

_____ Tubular shaft of a long bone

_____ Expanded ends of long bone

_____ Outer covering of a long bone

_____ Hollow region in the shaft

_____ Hyaline cartilage that covers the ends of the bone

_____ Connective tissue membrane that lines the shaft

5. Write the terms that fit the following descriptive phrases about the bone markings.

_____ Smooth, rounded articular surface

_____ Opening through a bone

_____ Smooth shallow depression

_____ Cavity or hollow space in a bone

_____ Smooth, flat articular surface

_____ Large blunt projections found on the femur

6. Write the terms that fit the following descriptive phrases about bone development and growth.

_____ Process of bone formation

_____ Cells that deposit bone matrix; bone-forming cells

_____ Mature bone cells located in lacunae

_____ Cells that destroy bone by removing bone matrix

_____ Type of ossification in most flat bones of the skull

_____ Bone development in which hyaline cartilage models are replaced by bone

_____ Region where long bones increase in length

_____ Cells in the periosteum that are responsible for increase in bone diameter

_____ Cells that hollow out the medullary cavity

_____ Type of ossification in most long bones of the body

7. How many named bones are in the complete skeleton? _____

How many named bones are in the axial skeleton? _____

How many named bones are in the appendicular skeleton? _____

Bones of the Axial Skeleton

1. Name the bones that form the cranium.

2. Name the bones that form the face.

3. For each of the following, name the bone of the skull that has the given feature.

   _____ Foramen magnum

   _____ Auditory meatus

   _____ Supraorbital foramen

   _____ Mastoid process

   _____ Optic foramen

   _____ Cribriform plate

   _____ Sella turcica

   _____ Ramus

4. What is the name of the U-shaped bone in the neck?

5. Write the terms that fit the following descriptive phrases about the axial skeleton.

   _____ First cervical vertebra

   _____ Vertebrae that articulate with ribs

   _____ Weight-bearing portion of a vertebra

   _____ Superior portion of the breastbone

   _____ Second cervical vertebra

   _____ Type of vertebrae in the neck

   _____ Vertebrae with heavy bodies and blunt processes

   _____ Another name for the breastbone

   _____ Cartilaginous pads between the vertebrae

6. State the number for each of the following.

   _____ True ribs   _____ Lumbar vertebrae

   _____ Cervical vertebrae   _____ Vertebrosternal ribs

   _____ False ribs   _____ Vertebral ribs

   _____ Thoracic vertebrae   _____ Vertebrochondral ribs

7. Identify the bones and selected features of the skull in the following diagram by placing the correct letter in the space provided by the listed labels. Then select a different color for each bone and use it to color the coding circles and the corresponding bone in the illustration.

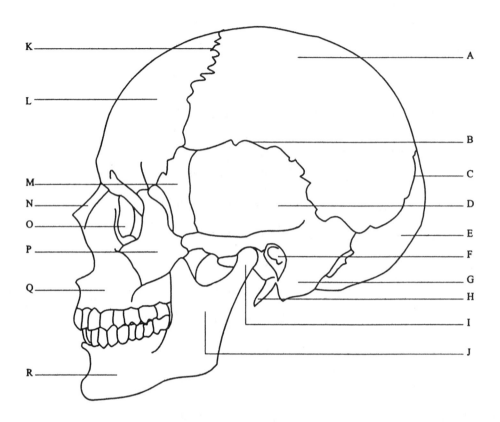

_____ Mandible ○

_____ Frontal ○

_____ Temporal ○

_____ Nasal ○

_____ Maxilla ○

_____ Occipital ○

_____ Zygomatic ○

_____ Sphenoid ○

_____ Lacrimal ○

_____ Parietal ○

_____ Ramus

_____ Coronal suture

_____ Mastoid process

_____ Mandibular condyle

_____ Styloid process

_____ Auditory meatus

_____ Squamosal suture

_____ Lambdoidal suture

Bones of the Appendicular Skeleton

1. Identify the bone or feature of the pectoral girdle and upper extremity that best fits each description given below.

_____ Anterior bone of the pectoral girdle

_____ Posterior bone of the pectoral girdle

_____ Bone that has an acromion and spine

_____ Large bone in the arm

_____ Bone on the lateral side of the forearm

_____ Bone on the medial side of the forearm

_____ Wrist bones

_____ Bones that form the palm of the hand

_____ Bones that form the fingers and toes

_____ Bone that articulates with the trochlea of humerus

_____ Bone that articulates with capitulum of humerus

_____ Projection on proximal end of ulna

2. Identify the bone or feature of the pelvic girdle and lower extremity that best fits each description given below.

_____ Three bones that fuse to form the os coxa

_____

_____

_____ Depression in the os coxa for the femoral head

_____ Portion of femur that articulates with tibia

_____ Bone on the medial side of the leg

_____ Bone on the lateral side of the leg

_____ Tarsal that forms the heel

_____ Tarsal that articulates with the tibia

_____ Bone in tendon anterior to femur and tibia

_____ Bone of axial skeleton articulating with os coxa

_____ Bone that has greater and lesser trochanters

3. Compare the pelvis in the male and female by completing the following table.

Feature	Male	Female
Pubic arch		
Pelvic inlet		
Pelvic cavity		

4. The portion of the pelvis between the flared wings of the ilium bones is called the
    _____ pelvis. The portion inferior to the pelvic brim is the
    _____ pelvis.

5. Identify the bones indicated on the anterior view of the skeleton, then color the axial skeleton red and the appendicular skeleton blue.

A. _____

B. _____

C. _____

D. _____

E. _____

F. _____

G. _____

H. _____

I. _____

J. _____

K. _____

L. _____

M. _____

N. _____

6. Identify the bones indicated on the posterior view of the skeleton, then color the axial skeleton red and the appendicular skeleton blue.

A. _____

B. _____

C. _____

D. _____

E. _____

F. _____

G. _____

H. _____

I. _____

J. _____

K. _____

L. _____

M. _____

N. _____

O. _____

P. _____

Q. _____

Fractures and Fracture Repair

1. Identify the following fractures by writing the name of the fracture on the line preceding the description.

_____ Broken bone protrudes through the skin

_____ Bone is crushed into multiple small pieces

_____ Break is at right angles to the bone's long axis

_____ Broken ends of the bone are not correctly aligned

_____ Bone is broken by twisting

2. Six-year-old Johnny Showman fell on his shoulder while at the playground. X-rays showed that the right clavicle was connected on the superior surface of the bone, but that the inferior surface was broken.

   a. Is this fracture open or closed?

   b. Is this fracture complete or incomplete?

   c. Arrange the events of fracture repair for Johnny's clavicle in the correct sequence by placing numbers 1-5 on the lines with 1 being the first event and 5 being the final event.

   _____ Bony callus

   _____ Fracture hematoma

   _____ Remodeling

   _____ Procallus

   _____ Fibrocartilaginous callus

Articulations

1. Indicate whether each of the following pertains to synarthroses, amphiarthroses, or diarthroses by writing the correct letter in the space provided before each descriptive phrase. S = synarthroses, A = amphiarthroses, D = diarthroses

   _____ Sutures   _____ Ball and socket

   _____ Slightly movable   _____ Ribs to sternum

   _____ Meniscus   _____ May have bursae

   _____ Immovable   _____ Joint capsule

   _____ Elbow and knee   _____ Symphysis pubis

REVIEW QUESTIONS

1. List five functions of the skeletal system.

2. What is the difference between compact bone and spongy bone? Where is each one located?

3. Give examples of long bones, short bones, flat bones, and irregular bones.

4. Draw and label the general features of a typical long bone.

5. What are osteoblasts, osteoclasts, and osteocytes?

6. How does intramembranous ossification differ from endochondral ossification?

7. Where in the bone do bones increase in length? How do they increase in diameter?

8. How many bones are in the axial skeleton? Appendicular skeleton?

9. Name the eight bones of the cranium.

10. Name the fourteen bones of the face.

11. What are auditory ossicles and where are they located?

12. What is unique about the hyoid bone?

13. What are the four curvatures of the vertebral column and when do they develop? What is their purpose?

14. What features are common to most vertebrae?

15. Identify at least two characteristics that are unique to cervical vertebrae, to thoracic vertebrae, and to lumbar vertebrae. How many of each type of vertebrae are there?

16. Where are the sacrum and coccyx located? What are their features?

17. What are the three parts of the sternum?

18. What is the difference between vertebral ribs, vertebrosternal ribs, and vertebrochondral ribs?

19. What bones are in the pectoral girdle?

20. Name the bones of the upper extremity and tell where they are located.

21. What three bones fuse to form an os coxa?

22. Define or describe each of the following: symphysis pubis, acetabulum, iliosacral joint, obturator foramen, iliac crest, greater sciatic notch, and ischial tuberosity.

23. What is the difference between the false pelvis and the true pelvis?

24. Name the bones of the lower extremity and tell where they are located.

25. What is the difference between open and closed fractures? Transverse and spiral fractures?

26. List the five steps of fracture repair in the sequence in which they occur.

27. What are three types of joints based on the amount of movement they permit? Give at least one example of each type.

28. List five structural features present in all synovial joints.

29. What are menisci and bursae? What is their purpose?

30. Name six different types of freely movable joints.

CHAPTER QUIZ

1. Match each of the following bones with its correct shape.

   _____ Carpals   A. long bone

   _____ Femur   B. short bone

   _____ Metatarsals   C. flat bone

   _____ Occipital   D. irregular bone

   _____ Phalanges

   _____ Sphenoid

   _____ Tarsals

   _____ Temporal

   _____ Tibia

   _____ Vertebrae

2. Match the following descriptions with the correct feature of a long bone.

   _____ Shaft   A. diaphysis

   _____ Hollow space in the center   B. endosteum

   _____ Expanded ends   C. epiphysis

   _____ Growth region   D. epiphyseal plate

   _____ Location of yellow marrow   E. medullary cavity

   _____ Location of red marrow   F. periosteum

   _____ Outer covering

   _____ Lining on inside of shaft

3. Indicate whether each of the following is part of the axial skeleton or part of the appendicular skeleton. Use X = axial and P = appendicular.

   _____ Calcaneus   _____ Mandible   _____ Scapula

   _____ Carpals   _____ Nasal conchae   _____ Sternum

   _____ Clavicle   _____ Ethmoid   _____ Occipital

   _____ Temporal   _____ Femur   _____ Os coxa

   _____ Tibia   _____ Humerus   _____ Patella

   _____ Ulna   _____ Lumbar vertebrae   _____ Ribs

   _____ Zygomatic   _____ Sacrum

4. Which one of the following is *not* a bone of the cranium? (a) ethmoid, (b) zygomatic, (c) temporal, (d) frontal, (e) sphenoid

5. Which one of the following is *not* a feature of thoracic vertebrae? (a) centrum or body, (b) long, sharp, spinous process, (c) articular facets for ribs, (d) transverse foramina; (e) vertebral canal

6. If the second item is a part of, or included in, the first, circle the T. If not, circle the F.

    T F Occipital bone   T F Scapula
          Foramen magnum   Acetabulum

    T F Sphenoid bone   T F Humerus
          Optic foramen   Coronoid process

    T F Os coxa   T F Os coxa
          Obturator foramen   Glenoid fossa

    T F Ethmoid bone   T F Ulna
          Inferior nasal conchae   Styloid process

7. Circle the earlier event in each of the following pairs of events in fracture repair.

    a. bony callus   procallus

    b. remodeling   fracture hematoma

    c. fibrocartilaginous callus   bony callus

    d. procallus   fracture hematoma

    e. bony callus   remodeling

8. Match the joints, descriptions, or features on the left with the appropriate term on the right.

    _____ Ball and socket joints   A. amphiarthrosis

    _____ Bursae   B. diarthrosis

    _____ Hinge joints   C. synarthrosis

    _____ Immovable joints

    _____ Intervertebral joints

    _____ Sutures

    _____ Symphysis pubis

    _____ Synovial membrane

USING CLINICAL KNOWLEDGE

1. Match the definitions on the left with the correct term from the column on the right by placing the corresponding letter in the space before the definition. Not all terms will be used.

_____   Shaft of a long bone

_____   Uric acid crystals develop within a joint causing acute inflammation

_____   Bone-forming cell

_____   Congenital deformity of the foot; clubfoot

_____   Ibuprofen

_____   Displacement of a bone from its joint with tearing of the articular cartilage

_____   Inflammation of a joint

_____   Twisting of a joint with injury to ligaments, tendons, muscles, blood vessels, nerves

_____   Acetaminophen

_____   Slightly movable joint

A. Amphiarthrosis

B. Arthritis

C. Diaphysis

D. Dislocation

E. Gout

F. NSAID

G. Osteoblast

H. Osteoclast

I. Sprain

J. Synarthrosis

K. Talipes

L. Tylenol

2. Write the meaning of the following abbreviations.

_____   DJD

_____   CTS

_____   ROM

_____   fx

_____   DIPJ

3. Spelling is important in scientific and medical applications because only one or two incorrect letters may change the meaning. All of the following words are from this chapter and are spelled incorrectly. Write the correct spelling in the space preceding the word.

_____   symarthrosis

_____   ileum

_____   carpel

_____   fibia

_____   falanges

4. Write the meaning of the underlined portion of each word on the line preceding the word.

_____ <u>kyph</u>osis

_____ hemato<u>poie</u>sis

_____ <u>spondyl</u>osis

_____ osteo<u>arthr</u>itis

_____ osteo<u>myel</u>itis

5. Using the following word parts, write words that fit the given definitions.

| -algia | chondr- | -ectomy | -pathy |
| arthr- | cost- | osteo- | phalang- |

_____ Excision of a finger or toe

_____ Pain in the ribs

_____ Disease of cartilage

_____ Surgical removal of a joint

_____ Any disease of both bones and joints

6. Separate each of the following words into its component parts, give the meaning of each part, then write the meaning of the entire word.

Osteoplasty:

_____

_____

_____

Ankylosis:

_____

_____

_____

FUN AND GAMES

The names of 50 bones and bone features are hidden in the word search puzzle below. They may read forward, backward, horizontally, vertically, or diagonally, but always in a straight line. See how many you can find.

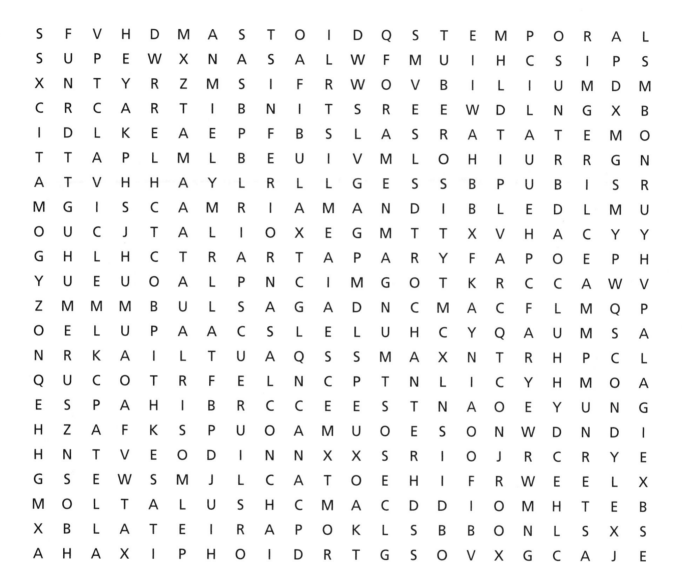

```
S  F  V  H  D  M  A  S  T  O  I  D  Q  S  T  E  M  P  O  R  A  L
S  U  P  E  W  X  N  A  S  A  L  W  F  M  U  I  H  C  S  I  P  S
X  N  T  Y  R  Z  M  S  I  F  R  W  O  V  B  I  L  I  U  M  D  M
C  R  C  A  R  T  I  B  N  I  T  S  R  E  E  W  D  L  N  G  X  B
I  D  L  K  E  A  E  P  F  B  S  L  A  S  R  A  T  A  T  E  M  O
T  T  A  P  L  M  L  B  E  U  I  V  M  L  O  H  I  U  R  R  G  N
A  T  V  H  H  A  Y  L  R  L  L  G  E  S  S  B  P  U  B  I  S  R
M  G  I  S  C  A  M  R  I  A  M  A  N  D  I  B  L  E  D  L  M  U
O  U  C  J  T  A  L  I  O  X  E  G  M  T  T  X  V  H  A  C  Y  Y
G  H  L  H  C  T  R  A  R  T  A  P  A  R  Y  F  A  P  O  E  P  H
Y  U  E  U  O  A  L  P  N  C  I  M  G  O  T  K  R  C  C  A  W  V
Z  M  M  M  B  U  L  S  A  G  A  D  N  C  M  A  C  F  L  M  Q  P
O  E  L  U  P  A  A  C  S  L  E  L  U  H  C  Y  Q  A  U  M  S  A
N  R  K  A  I  L  T  U  A  Q  S  S  M  A  X  N  T  R  H  P  C  L
Q  U  C  O  T  R  F  E  L  N  C  P  T  N  L  I  C  Y  H  M  O  A
E  S  P  A  H  I  B  R  C  C  E  E  S  T  N  A  O  E  Y  U  N  G
H  Z  A  F  K  S  P  U  O  A  M  U  O  E  S  O  N  W  D  N  D  I
H  N  T  V  E  O  D  I  N  N  X  X  S  R  I  O  J  R  C  R  Y  E
G  S  E  W  S  M  J  L  C  A  T  O  E  H  I  F  R  W  E  E  L  X
M  O  L  T  A  L  U  S  H  C  M  A  C  D  D  I  O  M  H  T  E  B
X  B  L  A  T  E  I  R  A  P  O  K  L  S  B  B  O  N  L  S  X  S
A  H  A  X  I  P  H  O  I  D  R  T  G  S  O  V  X  G  C  A  J  E
```

7

Muscular System

KEY TERMS

Actin
All-or-none principle
Antagonist
Insertion
Motor unit
Myosin
Neuromuscular junction
Neurotransmitter
Origin
Prime mover
Sarcomere
Synergist

BUILDING VOCABULARY

a-
act-
bi-
cep-
delt-
-desis
dia-
duct-
fasci-
flex-
-in
iso-
kinesi-
lemm-
masset-
metr-
myo-, mys-
phragm-
-rrhexis
sarco-

syn-
synov-
tetan-
ton-
troph-

CLINICAL TERMS

Cramp
Electromyography
Muscle biopsy
Muscular dystrophy
Myasthenia gravis
Myoparesis
Myopathy
Myorrhexis
Myositis
Repetitive stress disorder
Shin splint
Tenomyoplasty
Tenoplasty
Tenorraphy
Tic

CLINICAL ABBREVIATIONS

ACL
ad lib
amt
B/A
DTR
KD
LBP
LOS
MG
MS

CLINICAL ABBREVIATIONS *(cont'd)*

NYD   PTB
PMA   RSI
PRE

OUTLINE/OBJECTIVES

Characteristics and Functions of the Muscular System

- List the characteristics and functions of muscle tissue.
  — Skeletal muscle cells are cylindrical in shape, with many nuclei, and have striations. The muscles are attached to bones and produce movement under voluntary control.
  — Four characteristics of muscle tissue are excitability, contractility, extensibility, and elasticity.
  — Three functions of muscles are to produce movement, to maintain posture, and to produce heat necessary to maintain body temperature.

Structure of Skeletal Muscle

- Describe the structure of a skeletal muscle, including its connective tissue coverings.
  — A muscle consists of many muscle fibers or cells. Each muscle is surrounded by connective tissue called epimysium.
  — Inward extensions of the epimysium separate the muscle into bundles of fibers, called fasciculi, which are surrounded by perimysium.
  — Each individual muscle fiber is surrounded by connective tissue called endomysium.
  — The connective tissue coverings extend beyond the belly, or gaster, of the muscle to attach the muscle to bones or other muscles by way of tendons. The origin is the less movable end and the insertion is the more movable end.
- Identify the bands and lines that make up the striations on myofibers of skeletal muscle and relate these striations to actin and myosin.
  — A skeletal muscle fiber is a muscle cell with typical cellular organelles. The cell membrane is the sarcolemma, the cytoplasm is sarcoplasm, and the endoplasmic reticulum is called sarcoplasmic reticulum.
  — The sarcoplasm contains myofibrils that are made of still smaller units called myofilaments. Thick myofilaments are composed of the protein myosin, and thin myofilaments are formed from the protein actin.
  — The characteristic striations of skeletal muscle fibers (the A, I, and H bands) are due to the arrangement of the myosin and actin myofilaments. The Z and M lines are points of myofilament connections.
  — The A band is the entire length of the myosin filaments. The actin overlaps the myosin at the ends, making that region darker. The center of the A band, where there is only myosin, is the lighter H band. The I band is where there are only actin filaments.
  — A sarcomere is the functional, or contractile, unit of a myofibril. It extends from one Z line to the next Z line.
  — Skeletal muscles must be stimulated by a nerve before they can contract, therefore muscles have an abundant nerve supply; an abundant blood supply is necessary to deliver the nutrients and oxygen required for contraction.

Contraction of Skeletal Muscle

- Describe the sequence of events involved in the contraction of a skeletal muscle fiber.

— A neuromuscular junction is the region where an axon terminal of a motor neuron is closely associated with a muscle fiber. Acetylcholine, a neurotransmitter released by the motor neuron, diffuses across the synaptic cleft to stimulate the sarcolemma of a muscle fiber. Acetylcholinesterase is an enzyme that inactivates acetylcholine to prevent continued contraction from a single impulse.

— When a muscle fiber is stimulated, an impulse travels down the sarcolemma into a T tubule, which releases calcium ions from the sarcoplasmic reticulum. Calcium alters the configuration of actin and energizes myosin by breaking down ATP.

— Cross-bridges form between the actin and myosin, and the energy from the ATP results in a power stroke that pulls actin toward the center of the myosin myofilaments. This shortens the length of the sarcomere.

— When stimulation at the neuromuscular junction stops, calcium returns to the sarcoplasmic reticulum, and actin and myosin resume their noncontracting positions.

— The minimum stimulus necessary to cause muscle fiber contraction is a threshold, or liminal, stimulus. A lesser stimulus is subthreshold, or subliminal.

— Individual muscle fibers contract according to the all-or-none principle. If a threshold stimulus is applied, the fiber will contract; a greater stimulus does not create a more forceful contraction. If the stimulus is subthreshold, the fiber does not contract at all.

• Compare the different types of muscle contractions.

— Whole muscles show varying strengths of contraction due to motor unit and wave summation. A motor unit is a single motor neuron and all the muscle fibers it stimulates. Contraction strength of a whole muscle can be increased in response to increased load (stimulus) by stimulating more motor units, thus multiple motor unit summation.

— A muscle twitch, the response to a single stimulus, shows a lag phase, a contraction phase, and a relaxation phase. If a second stimulus of the same intensity as the first is applied before the relaxation phase is complete, a second contraction, stronger than the first, results. Repeated stimulation of the same strength that results in stronger contractions is called multiple wave summation.

— Rapid repeated stimulation that allows no relaxation results in a smooth sustained contraction that is stronger than the contraction from a single stimulus of the same intensity. This is tetanus, a form of multiple wave summation. This is the usual form of muscle contraction.

— Treppe is the staircase effect that is evidenced when repeated stimuli of the same strength produce successively stronger contractions. This is due to changes in the cellular environment.

— Muscle tone refers to the continued state of partial contraction in muscles. It is important in maintaining posture and body temperature.

— Isotonic contractions produce movement but muscle tension remains constant. Isometric contractions increase muscle tension but do not produce movement. Most body movements involve both types of contractions.

• Describe how energy is provided for muscle contraction and how oxygen debt occurs.

— In muscle contraction, energy is needed for the power stroke, detachment of myosin heads, and active transport of calcium.

— ATP provides the initial energy for muscle contraction. The ATP supply is replenished by creatine phosphate.

— When muscles are actively contracting for extended periods of time, glucose becomes the primary energy source to produce more ATP.

— When adequate oxygen is available, glucose is metabolized by aerobic respiration to produce ATP. If adequate oxygen is not available, the mechanism for producing ATP from glucose is anaerobic respiration. Aerobic respiration produces nearly 20 times more ATP per glucose than the anaerobic pathway, but anaerobic respiration occurs at a faster rate.

— Oxygen debt occurs when there is an accumulation of lactic acid from anaerobic respiration. Additional oxygen from continued labored breathing is needed to repay the debt and restore resting conditions.
- Describe and illustrate movements accomplished by the contraction of skeletal muscle.
  — A prime mover, or agonist, has the major role in producing a specific movement; a synergist assists the prime mover; an antagonist opposes a particular movement.
  — Descriptive terms used to depict particular movements include flexion, extension, hyperextension, dorsiflexion, plantar flexion, abduction, adduction, rotation, supination, pronation, circumduction, inversion, and eversion.

Skeletal Muscle Groups

- Locate, identify, and describe the actions of the major muscles of the axial skeleton.
  — Muscles of facial expression include the frontalis, orbicularis oris, orbicularis oculi, buccinator, and zygomaticus.
  — Chewing muscles are called muscles of mastication and include the masseter and temporalis.
  — Neck muscles include the sternocleidomastoid, which flexes the neck, and the trapezius, which extends the neck.
  — Muscles that act on the vertebral column include the erector spinae group and the deep back muscles. The erector spinae form a large muscle mass that extends from the sacrum to the skull on each side of the vertebral column. The deep back muscles are short muscles that occupy the space between the spinous and transverse processes of adjacent vertebrae.
  — Muscles of the thoracic wall are involved in the process of breathing. These include the intercostal muscles and the diaphragm.
  — Abdominal wall muscles include the external oblique, internal oblique, transversus abdominis, and rectus abdominis. These muscles provide strength and support to the abdominal wall.
  — Pelvic floor muscles form a covering for the pelvic outlet and provide support for the pelvic viscera. The superficial muscles form the urogenital diaphragm, and the deeper muscles, the levator ani, form the pelvic diaphragm.
- Locate, identify, and describe the actions of the major muscles of the appendicular skeleton.
  — The trapezius and serratus anterior muscles attach the scapula to the axial skeleton and move the scapula.
  — The pectoralis major, latissimus dorsi, deltoid, and rotator cuff muscles insert on the humerus and move the arm.
  — The triceps brachii, in the posterior compartment of the arm, extends the forearm. The biceps brachii and brachialis muscles, in the anterior compartment, flex the forearm.
  — The brachioradialis muscle, primarily located in the forearm, flexes and supinates the forearm.
  — Most of the muscles that are located on the forearm act on the wrist, hand, or fingers.
  — The gluteus maximus, gluteus medius, gluteus minimus, and tensor fasciae latae muscles abduct the thigh. The iliopsoas, an anterior muscle, flexes the thigh.
  — The muscles in the medial compartment include the adductor longus, adductor brevis, adductor magnus, and gracilis muscles. These muscles adduct the thigh.
  — The quadriceps femoris muscle group, located in the anterior compartment of the thigh, straightens the leg at the knee.
  — The sartorius muscle, a long straplike muscle on the anterior surface of the thigh, flexes and medially rotates the leg.
  — The hamstring muscles, in the posterior compartment of the thigh, are antagonists to the quadriceps femoris muscle group.

— The principal muscle in the anterior compartment of the leg is the tibialis anterior, which dorsiflexes the foot.

— Contraction of the peroneus muscles, in the lateral compartment of the leg, everts the foot.

— The gastrocnemius and soleus form the bulky mass of the posterior compartment of the leg. These muscles plantar flex the foot.

LEARNING EXERCISES

Characteristics and Functions of the Muscular System

1. Match the correct type of muscle tissue with each descriptive word or phrase.

    _____   Striated and involuntary   A. skeletal

    _____   Spindle-shaped fibers   B. visceral

    _____   Multinucleated and cylindrical   C. cardiac

    _____   Found in blood vessels

    _____   Found in the heart

2. List four characteristics of muscle tissue that relate to its functions.

    (a)

    (b)

    (c)

    (d)

3. Three functions of muscle contraction are:

    (a)

    (b)

    (c)

Structure of Skeletal Muscle

1. Write the terms that fit the following descriptive phrases in the space provided.

    _____   More movable attachment of a muscle

    _____   Covering around an individual muscle fiber

    _____   Protein in thick myofilaments

    _____   Bundle of fibers surrounded by perimysium

    _____   Less movable attachment of a muscle

_____ Broad, flat sheet of tendon

_____ Cell membrane of a muscle cell

_____ Protein in thin myofilaments

_____ Unit of muscle between Z lines

_____ Type of myofilament in the I band

2. Muscle fibers must be stimulated before they can contract, therefore they have an abundant _____. The blood supply delivers _____ and _____ for contraction.

Contraction of Skeletal Muscle

1. Arrange the following events of muscle contraction in the correct sequence by writing a number 1 before the first event, number 2 before the second event, and so forth until the 8 events have been numbered correctly.

_____ Energized myosin heads attach to actin

_____ Acetylcholine is released into synaptic cleft

_____ Power stroke pulls actin toward center of A band

_____ Calcium reacts with troponin and exposes binding sites on actin

_____ Acetylcholine reacts with receptors on sarcolemma

_____ Nerve impulse reaches axon terminal

_____ Calcium ions are released from the sarcoplasmic reticulum

_____ Impulse travels into the T tubules

2. Write the terms that match the statements in the spaces provided.

_____ Minimum stimulus that causes contraction

_____ Principle by which muscle fibers contract

_____ Stimulus insufficient to cause contraction

_____ Single neuron and muscle fibers it stimulates

_____ Increases contraction strength in a muscle

_____ Sustained contraction due to rapid stimuli

_____ Staircase effect due to a series of stimuli

_____ Continued state of partial muscle contraction

_____ Muscle contraction with constant tension

_____ Muscle contraction with changing tension

3. Write the terms that match the statements in the spaces provided.

_____   Immediate source of energy for contraction

_____   Stored in muscle to regenerate ATP

_____   Molecule that stores oxygen in muscle

_____   Acid that accumulates with lack of oxygen

_____   Products of aerobic breakdown of pyruvic acid

4. The muscle that has a primary role in providing a movement is called the
_____. Muscles that assist this muscle are called
_____ and muscles that oppose the movement are called
_____.

5. Match the type of muscle movement with the description. Not all responses will be used.

_____ Extension of foot to stand on tiptoes   A. flexion

_____ Movement of arm toward the midline   B. extension

_____ Straightening the arm at the elbow   C. hyperextension

_____ Turning the palm of the hand forward   D. dorsiflexion

_____ Turning the head from side to side   E. plantar flexion

_____ Moving elbow to put hand on shoulder   F. abduction

_____ Turning the sole of foot inward   G. adduction

_____ Spreading the fingers apart   H. rotation

_____ Tilting head backward   I. supination

_____ Drawing circles on chalkboard   J. pronation

                                                     K. circumduction

                                                     L. inversion

                                                     M. eversion

Skeletal Muscle Groups

1. Write the type of muscle feature that is indicated by each of the following muscle names: size, shape, direction of fibers, location, number of origins, origin/insertion, or action.

_____   Adductor

_____   Rectus

_____   Maximus

_____   Gluteus

_____ Deltoid

_____ Biceps

_____ Brachioradialis

_____ Pectoralis

2. Write the name of the muscle that matches each action.

_____ Raises the eyebrows

_____ Closes and puckers the lips

_____ Raises the mandible in chewing (2)

_____

_____ Closes the eye in squinting

_____ Flexes neck so the chin drops

_____ Primary muscle in inspiration

_____ Anterior muscle that adducts and flexes arm

_____ Posterior muscle that adducts arm

_____ Abducts the arm

_____ Extends the forearm

_____ Has two heads and flexes forearm

_____ Inserts on ulna and flexes forearm

_____ Inserts on femur; flexes thigh

_____ Synergist of iliopsoas

_____ Antagonist of iliopsoas

_____ Group that adducts thigh

_____ Group that extends the leg

_____ Muscles that flex the leg (3)

_____

_____

_____ Muscles that plantar flex the foot (2)

_____

_____ Antagonist of the gastrocnemius

3. Identify the muscles indicated on the following diagrams.

A. _____

B. _____

C. _____

D. _____

E. _____

F. _____

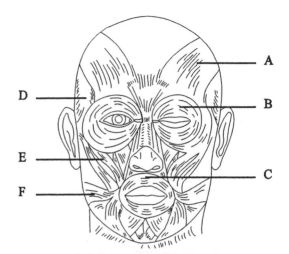

G. _____

H. _____

I. _____

J. _____

K. _____

L. _____

M. _____

N. _____

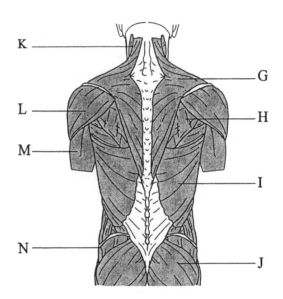

4. Identify the muscles indicated on the following diagrams.

A. _____

B. _____

C. _____

D. _____

E. _____

F. _____

G. _____

H. _____

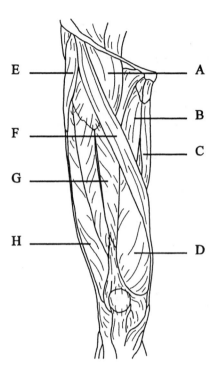

I. _____

J. _____

K. _____

L. _____

M. _____

N. _____

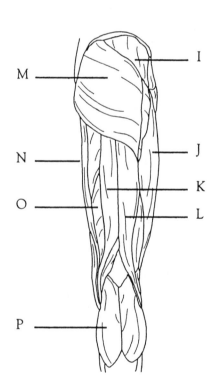

REVIEW QUESTIONS

1. How does skeletal muscle differ from visceral muscle in terms of appearance?

2. What are four characteristics of muscle tissue?

3. Skeletal muscles produce movement. What are two other functions of skeletal muscle tissue?

4. What are the endomysium, epimysium, and perimysium?

5. What is the term used to designate the more movable attachment of a muscle?

6. What protein is found in the thick myofilaments? What protein is found in the thin myofilaments?

7. What type of myofilaments makes up the (a) A band; (b) I band; (c) H band?

8. What designates the region between two successive Z lines?

9. Why does skeletal muscle need an abundant blood and nerve supply?

10. What is the neurotransmitter that is released at the neuromuscular junction to stimulate the muscle fiber?

11. What changes occur in the configuration of actin that allow cross-bridges to form between the actin and myosin? What ion is responsible for the changes?

12. Write a sentence that defines the all-or-none principle.

13. What is a motor unit?

14. What is the difference between multiple motor unit summation and multiple wave summation?

15. What type of muscle contraction is responsible for producing movement?

16. What are the immediate, intermediate, and long-term sources of energy for muscle contraction?

17. What organic molecule accumulates when oxygen debt occurs?

18. How do synergists and antagonists relate to the prime mover in a muscle action?

19. What is the opposite of (a) flexion; (b) abduction; (c) pronation; (d) dorsiflexion?

20. Identify the (a) two circular muscles of the face; (b) muscle the elevates the corner of the mouth to form a smile; (c) two muscles that close the jaw when chewing; (d) muscle in the neck that is antagonistic to the sternocleidomastoid.

21. Name the four muscles that constitute the anterolateral abdominal wall.

22. What muscle is antagonistic to the external intercostal muscles?

23. Name two muscles that move the shoulder.

24. What is the function of the (a) deltoid; (b) pectoralis major; (c) latissimus dorsi?

25. Name (a) two muscles that are synergists of the biceps brachii; (b) one muscle that is an antagonist of the biceps brachii.

26. Name the muscle that is (a) a synergist of the iliopsoas; (b) an antagonist of the iliopsoas.

27. Identify four muscles that adduct the thigh.

28. What three muscles make up the hamstrings? What is their function?

29. What four muscles make up the quadriceps femoris? What is their function?

30. What muscle that moves the leg is the longest muscle in the body?

31. What two muscle tendons join to form the Achilles tendon?

32. What muscle is in the anterior compartment of the leg and dorsiflexes the foot?

CHAPTER QUIZ

1. Place an X before the characteristics that pertain to skeletal muscle tissue.

   _____ Responds to a stimulus

   _____ Multinucleated

   _____ Centrally located nucleus

   _____ Striations

   _____ Intercalated disks

   _____ Located in the wall of the stomach

2. The connective tissue covering around a fasciculus of skeletal muscle fibers is called
   _____.

3. The fixed, or stable, end of a muscle is called the _____.

4. The region of a myofibril that has only actin filaments is the (a) A band; (b) I band; (c) H band; (d) M band; (e) Z band.

5. Name the following:

   _____ Cell membrane of a muscle cell

   _____ Neurotransmitter at neuromuscular junction

   _____ Protein in thick filaments

   _____ Molecule that accumulates in anaerobic respiration

   _____ Storage site for calcium ions

   _____ Immediate energy source for contraction

   _____ Type of contraction that produces movement

   _____ Muscle response to a single stimulus

   _____ A type of multiple wave summation

   _____ Staircase effect of contraction

6. Which of the following pairs of terms does *not* represent opposite actions? (a) flexion/extension; (b) rotation/pronation; (c) inversion/eversion; (d) abduction/adduction; (e) dorsiflexion/plantar flexion

7. When you bend the elbow to touch your right shoulder with your right hand, the action at the elbow is (a) abduction; (b) supination; (c) circumduction; (d) flexion; (e) inversion.

8. Match the following descriptions with the appropriate muscle.

_____ Closes the jaw in mastication

_____ Elevates the corner of the mouth in smiling

_____ Extends the head; holds the head upright

_____ Long, straight muscle of the anterior abdomen

_____ Moves the scapula

_____ Adducts the arm

_____ Antagonist of the latissimus dorsi

_____ Inserts on the radius

_____ Antagonist of the biceps brachii

_____ Located in medial compartment of thigh

_____ Most superficial and lateral muscle in the thigh

_____ Long straplike muscle that flexes thigh and leg

_____ Muscle group that extends the leg at the knee

_____ Located in the posterior compartment of the leg

_____ Muscle group that flexes the leg at the knee

_____ Muscle that allows you to "walk on your heels"

A. adductor longus

B. biceps brachii

C. deltoid

D. gastrocnemius

E. hamstrings

F. masseter

G. pectoralis major

H. quadriceps femoris

I. rectus abdominis

J. sartorius

K. serratus anterior

L. tensor fasciae latae

M. tibialis anterior

N. trapezius

O. triceps brachii

P. zygomaticus

USING CLINICAL KNOWLEDGE

1. Match the definitions on the left with the correct term from the column on the right by placing the corresponding letter in the space before the definition. Not all terms will be used.

_____	Slight muscle paralysis	A. Cramp
_____	Inflammation of a fascia	B. Fasciitis
_____	Muscle disease	C. Myoparesis
_____	Inflammation of a muscle	D. Myopathy
_____	Suture of a tendon	E. Myorrhexis
_____	Spasmodic involuntary twitching of a muscle that is normally under voluntary control	F. Myositis
		G. Synergist
_____	Painful involuntary muscle spasm	H. Tenomyoplasty
		I. Tenorraphy
		J. Tic

2. Write the meaning of the following abbreviations.

_____ ACL

_____ LOS

_____ RSI

_____ PMA

_____ DTR

3. Spelling is important in scientific and medical applications because only one or two incorrect letters may change the meaning. For each of the following pairs of words, circle the one that is spelled correctly.

myosin	mysin
myorexis	myorrhexis
diaphram	diaphragm
acetylcholine	acetilcoline
gastronemius	gastrocnemius
aponeurosis	aponurosis

4. Use these word parts to write terms that fit the given definitions.

-desis   myo-   -plasty   -tomy
fasci-   -pathy   -rraphy

_____   Any abnormal condition of skeletal muscle

_____   Suturing of torn fascia

_____   Surgical incision into, or division of, a muscle

_____   Suture of a fascia to skeletal attachment

_____   Surgical repair of a muscle

5. Ima Student's primary care practitioner prescribed a central-acting muscle relaxant to decrease some muscle spasms.

   a.   How do these drugs work?

   b.   List at least four side effects that may occur with these muscle relaxants.

FUN AND GAMES

The object of this puzzle is to accumulate as many points as possible for the words you select as answers for the clues. To do the puzzle, answer each clue with a **single** word and write that word in the space by the clue. Each letter of the alphabet is assigned point values as indicated. Using these point values, add up your score for each answer. Each clue has more than one possible answer and you should try to choose the one that gives the highest point value. Finally, add the ten individual scores to get your total score for the puzzle. For fair play, use single word answers only and avoid answers, such as orbicularis oris and pectoralis major, that contain two words. Try competing with your classmates to see who can get the highest score! Have fun!!

A = 1	B = 2	C = 2	D = 2	E = 1	F = 3	G = 3
H = 3	I = 1	J = 5	K = 4	L = 2	M = 2	N = 1
O = 1	P = 3	Q = 5	R = 1	S = 1	T = 1	U = 1
V = 4	W = 4	X = 5	Y = 3	Z = 5		

Clue	*Single Word Answer*	*Points*
1. A characteristic of muscle tissue	_____	_____
2. Connective tissue coverings associated with muscles and muscle fibers	_____	_____
3. A contractile protein in muscle	_____	_____
4. Attachment of a muscle	_____	_____
5. Phase of a muscle twitch	_____	_____
6. Descriptive term to depict a particular movement	_____	_____
7. Word in muscle name that describes direction of fibers	_____	_____
8. A muscle of facial expression	_____	_____
9. A muscle that moves the brachium	_____	_____
10. A muscle in posterior compartment of the leg	_____	_____

8

Nervous System

KEY TERMS

Action potential
Brain stem
Cerebellum
Cerebrum
Diencephalon
Myelin
Neurilemma
Saltatory conduction
Synapse
Threshold stimulus

BUILDING VOCABULARY

af-
algesi-
astro-
contra-
corpor-
dendr-
ef-
encephal-
esthes-
-fer-
gangli-
gli-
gloss-
idio-
lemm-
-lepsy
-mania
mening-
narc-
neur-
peri-
pharyng-

phas-
pleg-
plex-
schiz-
somn-
suic-

CLINICAL TERMS

Amyotrophic lateral sclerosis
Bell's palsy
Cerebral concussion
Cerebral contusion
Cerebral palsy
Cerebrovascular accident
Computed tomography
Electroencephalography
Magnetic resonance imaging
Multiple sclerosis
Positron emission tomography
Reye's syndrome
Shingles
Tic douloureux
Transient ischemic attack

CLINICAL ABBREVIATIONS

ADD
ADHD
ALS
ANS
CNS
CSF
CSM
CT
CVA

115

CLINICAL ABBREVIATIONS *(cont'd)*

EEG	PNS
ICP	SCI
OCD	SNS
PEG	

OUTLINE/OBJECTIVES

Functions and Organization of the Nervous System

- Outline the organization and functions of the nervous system.
  - The nervous system is divided into the central nervous system and the peripheral nervous system.
  - The peripheral nervous system consists of an afferent (sensory) division and an efferent (motor) division.
  - The efferent (motor) division is divided into the somatic nervous system and the autonomic nervous system.
  - The autonomic nervous system is further divided into the sympathetic and parasympathetic divisions.
  - The activities of the nervous system can be grouped into sensory, integrative, and motor functions.

Nerve Tissue

- Compare the structure and functions of neurons and neuroglia.
  - Neurons are the nerve cells that transmit impulses. They are amitotic.
  - The three components of a neuron are a cell body or soma, one or more dendrites, and a single axon.
  - Many neurons are surrounded by segmented myelin. The gaps in the myelin are the nodes of Ranvier. An outer covering, the neurilemma, plays a role in nerve regeneration.
  - Axons terminate in telodendria, which have synaptic bulbs on the distal end.
  - Functionally, neurons are classified as afferent (sensory), efferent (motor), or interneurons (association).
  - Neuroglia support, protect, and nourish the neurons. They are capable of mitosis.
  - Neuroglia cells include astrocytes, microglia, ependyma, oligodendrocytes, neurolemmocytes, and satellite cells.

Nerve Impulses

- Describe the sequence of events that lead to an action potential when the cell membrane is stimulated and how the impulse is conducted along the length of a neuron.
  - Excitability, the ability to respond to a stimulus, and conductivity, the ability to transmit an impulse, are two functional characteristics of neurons.
  - The cell membrane of a non-conducting neuron is polarized with an abundance of sodium ions outside the cell and an abundance of potassium and negatively charged proteins inside the cell. The inside of the membrane is approximately 70 millivolts negative to the outside.
  - In response to a stimulus, the cell membrane becomes permeable to sodium ions, so they rapidly enter the cell and depolarize the membrane. Continued sodium ion diffusion causes reverse polarization.

- — After reverse polarization, the membrane becomes impermeable to sodium and permeable to potassium. Potassium diffuses out of the cell to repolarize the membrane.
- — The action potential is a result of depolarization, reverse polarization, and repolarization of the cell membrane.
- — After the action potential, active transport mechanisms move sodium out of the cell and potassium into the cell to restore resting conditions.
- — A threshold stimulus is the minimum stimulus necessary to start an action potential. A weaker stimulus is subthreshold.
- — An action potential at a given point stimulates depolarization at an adjacent point to create a propagated action potential, or nerve impulse, that continues along the entire length of the neuron.
- — Saltatory conduction occurs in myelinated fibers where the action potential "jumps" from node to node.
- — The refractory period is the time during which the cell membrane is recovering from depolarization; absolute refractory period is the time during which the membrane is permeable to sodium ions and cannot respond to a second stimulus no matter how strong; relative refractory period is roughly comparable to the time when the membrane is permeable to potassium. During this time, it takes a stronger than normal stimulus to initiate an action potential.
- — If a threshold stimulus is applied, an action potential is generated and propagated along the entire length of the neuron at maximum strength and speed for the existing conditions.
- Describe the structure of a synapse and how an impulse is conducted from one neuron to another across the synapse.
  - — A synapse, the region of communication between two neurons, consists of a synaptic knob, a synaptic cleft, and the postsynaptic membrane.
  - — At the synapse, a neurotransmitter, such as acetylcholine, diffuses across the synaptic cleft and reacts with receptors on the postsynaptic membrane.
  - — In excitatory transmission, the reaction between the neurotransmitter and receptor depolarizes the postsynaptic membrane and initiates an action potential.
  - — In inhibitory transmission, the reaction between the neurotransmitter and receptor opens the potassium channels and hyperpolarizes the membrane, which makes it more difficult to generate an action potential.
  - — In a single series circuit, a single neuron synapses with another neuron; in a divergence circuit, a single neuron synapses with multiple neurons; and in a convergence circuit, several presynaptic neurons synapse with a single postsynaptic neuron.
- List the five basic components of a reflex arc.
  - — The reflex arc is a type of conduction pathway and represents the functional unit of the nervous system.
  - — A reflex arc utilizes a receptor, sensory neuron, center, motor neuron, and effector.

Central Nervous System

- Describe the three layers of meninges around the central nervous system.
  - — The brain and spinal cord are covered by three layers of connective tissue membranes called meninges.
  - — The outer layer of the meninges is the dura mater, the middle layer is the arachnoid, and the inner layer is the pia mater.
  - — The subarachnoid space, between the arachnoid and pia mater, contains blood vessels and cerebrospinal fluid.
- Locate and identify the major regions of the brain and describe their functions.
  - — The largest portion of the brain is the cerebrum, which is divided by a longitudinal fissure into two cerebral hemispheres. These are connected by a band of white fibers called the corpus callosum. The surface is marked by gyri separated by sulci.

— Each cerebral hemisphere is divided into frontal, parietal, occipital, and temporal lobes, and an insula.
— The outer surface of the cerebrum is the cerebral cortex and is composed of gray matter. This surrounds the white matter, which consists of myelinated nerve fibers. Basal ganglia are regions of gray matter scattered throughout the white matter.
— The somatosensory area is the postcentral gyrus in the parietal lobe; the sensory area for vision is in the occipital lobe; the area for hearing is in the temporal lobe; the olfactory area is in the temporal lobe; and the sensory area for taste is in the parietal lobe.
— The somatomotor area is the precentral gyrus in the frontal lobe.
— Association areas analyze, interpret, and integrate information. They are scattered throughout the cortex.
— The diencephalon is nearly surrounded by the cerebral cortex. It includes the thalamus, hypothalamus, and epithalamus.
— The largest region of the diencephalon is the thalamus, which serves as a relay station for sensory impulses going to the cerebral cortex.
— The hypothalamus is a small region below the thalamus. It plays a key role in maintaining homeostasis.
— The epithalamus is the superior portion of the diencephalon, and the pineal gland extends from its posterior margin.
— The brain stem is the region between the diencephalon and the spinal cord.
— The midbrain, the most superior portion of the brain stem, includes the cerebral peduncles and corpora quadrigemina. The midbrain contains voluntary motor tracts, and visual and auditory reflex centers.
— The pons is the middle portion of the brain stem. It contains the pneumotaxic and apneustic areas that help regulate breathing movements.
— The medulla oblongata is inferior to the pons and is continuous with the spinal cord. It contains ascending and descending nerve fibers. It also contains the vital cardiac, vasomotor, and respiratory centers.
— The cerebellum consists of two hemispheres connected by a central region called the vermis. A thin layer of gray matter, the cortex, surrounds the white matter.
— Cerebellar peduncles connect the cerebellum to other parts of the central nervous system (CNS).
— The cerebellum is a motor area that coordinates skeletal muscle activity and is important in maintaining muscle tone, posture, and balance.
• Trace the flow of cerebrospinal fluid from its origin in the ventricles to its return to the blood.
— Four interconnected cavities, called ventricles, contain cerebrospinal fluid within the brain.
— Cerebrospinal fluid (CSF) is formed as a filtrate from the blood in the choroid plexus in the ventricles.
— CSF moves from the lateral ventricles, through the interventricular foramen to the third ventricle, through the cerebral aqueduct to the fourth ventricle. From the fourth ventricle, it enters the subarachnoid space and filters through arachnoid granulations into the dural sinuses and is returned to the blood.
• Describe the structure and functions of the spinal cord.
— The spinal cord begins at the foramen magnum, as a continuation of the medulla oblongata, and extends to the first lumbar vertebra.
— The central core of the spinal cord is gray matter, which is divided into regions called dorsal, lateral, and ventral horns. The white matter, which surrounds the gray matter, is divided into dorsal, lateral, and ventral funiculi, or columns.
— The spinal cord is a conduction pathway and a reflex center.
— Ascending tracts in the spinal cord conduct sensory impulses to the brain. Conduction pathways that carry motor impulses from the brain to effectors are descending tracts.

Peripheral Nervous System

- Describe the structure of a nerve.
  - The cranial and spinal nerves form the peripheral nervous system. Nerves are classified as sensory, motor, or mixed, depending on the types of fibers they contain.
  - Nerves are bundles of nerve fibers.
  - Each individual nerve fiber is covered by endoneurium.
  - A bundle of nerve fibers, surrounded by perineurium, is called a fasciculus.
  - A nerve contains many fasciculi collected together and surrounded by epineurium.
- List the twelve cranial nerves and state the function of each one.
  - Twelve pairs of cranial nerves emerge from the inferior surface of the brain. Cranial nerves are designated by name and by Roman numerals.
  - Names of the cranial nerves are: olfactory (I), optic (II), oculomotor (III), trochlear (IV), trigeminal (V), abducens (VI), facial (VII), vestibulocochlear (VIII), glossopharyngeal (IX), vagus (X), accessory (XI), and hypoglossal (XII).
- Discuss spinal nerves and the plexuses they form.
  - All spinal nerves are mixed nerves. They are connected to the spinal cord by dorsal roots, which have only sensory fibers, and ventral roots, which have only motor fibers.
  - The 31 pairs of spinal nerves are grouped according to the region of the cord from which they originate. There are 8 cervical nerves, 12 thoracic nerves, 5 lumbar nerves, 5 sacral nerves, and 1 coccygeal nerve.
  - In all but the thoracic region, the main portions of the spinal nerves form complex networks called plexuses. Named nerves exit the plexuses to supply specific regions of the body.
- Compare the structural and functional differences between the somatic efferent pathways and the autonomic nervous system (ANS).
  - The ANS is a visceral efferent system that innervates smooth muscle, cardiac muscle, and glands.
  - An autonomic pathway consists of two neurons. A preganglionic neuron leaves the CNS and synapses with a postganglionic neuron in an autonomic ganglion.
- Distinguish between the sympathetic and parasympathetic divisions of the autonomic nervous system in terms of structure, function, and neurotransmitters.
  - The sympathetic division is also called the thoracolumbar division because its preganglionic neurons originate in the thoracic and lumbar regions of the spinal cord. It is an energy-expending system that prepares the body for emergency or stressful conditions.
  - The parasympathetic division, also called the craniosacral division because its preganglionic neurons originate in the brain and the sacral region of the spinal cord, is an energy-conserving system that is most active when the body is in a normal relaxed condition.

LEARNING EXERCISES

Functions of the Nervous System

1. The activities of the nervous system are grouped into three functional categories. These are _____, _____, and _____.

Organization of the Nervous System

1. The two components of the central nervous system are the _____ and _____.

2. The two divisions of the peripheral nervous system are the _____, or sensory division, and the _____, or motor division.

3. The autonomic nervous system is a part of the _____ division of the peripheral nervous system.

Nerve Tissue

1. Write the terms that fit the following descriptive phrases about neurons.

_____ Process that conducts impulses toward the cell body

_____ Fatty substance around some axons

_____ Neurons that carry impulses toward the CNS

_____ Gaps in the fatty substance around axons

_____ Neurons entirely within the CNS

_____ Conducts impulses away from the cell body

_____ Has important role in nerve fiber regeneration

2. Label the following diagram of a neuron.

   A. _____

   B. _____

   C. _____

   D. _____

   E. _____

   F. _____

   G. _____

   H. _____

   I. _____

3. Write the name of the neuroglial cell that best fits each descriptive phrase.

_____ Binds blood vessels to nerves

_____ Phagocytic

_____ Produces myelin within the CNS

_____ Produces myelin within the PNS

_____ Facilitates circulation of CSF

_____ Supports cell bodies within ganglia

Nerve Impulses

1. Two functional characteristics of neurons are _____ and

_____ .

2. At rest, the outside of a neuron is _____ (charge) and has
a higher concentration of _____ ions relative to the inside.
A stimulus changes the permeability of the membrane and it depolarizes. During depolarization, _____ ions diffuse into the cell. This creates an
_____ potential, or nerve impulse. During repolarization,
_____ ions diffuse out of the cell. At the conclusion of the
_____ , the _____ pump restores
the ionic conditions of a resting membrane. The minimum stimulus required to initiate a nerve
impulse is called a _____ stimulus.

3. Arrange the following numbered elements of a reflex arc in the correct sequence, beginning
with the application of a stimulus, by writing the numbers in the appropriate order on the line
provided. 1) Axon of interneuron; 2) Axon of motor neuron; 3) Axon of sensory neuron; 4) Cell
body of interneuron; 5) Cell body of motor neuron; 6) Cell body of sensory neuron; 7) Dendrite
of interneuron; 8) Dendrite of motor neuron; 9) Dendrite of sensory neuron; 10) Effector;
11) Sensory receptor; 12) Synapse between interneuron and motor neuron; 13) Synapse
between interneuron and sensory neuron

____ ____ ____ ____ ____ ____ ____ ____ ____ ____ ____ ____ ____

4. Match each of the following terms with the correct descriptive phrase.

A. convergence   D. inhibitory   G. refractory period
B. divergence   E. neurotransmitter   H. saltatory
C. excitatory   F. reflex arc   I. synapse

_____ Rapid conduction from node to node

_____ Region of communication between two neurons

_____ Diffuses across synaptic cleft

_____ Time during which a neuron is recovering from depolarization

_____ Synaptic transmission that initiates an impulse on the postsynaptic membrane

_____ Functional unit of the nervous system

_____ Single neuron synapses with multiple neurons

_____ Synaptic transmission that makes it more difficult to generate an impulse

_____ Several neurons synapse with a single postsynaptic neuron

Central Nervous System

1. Arrange the following spaces and CNS coverings in the correct sequence by placing numbers 1-6 on the lines provided. Use 1 for the **outermost** and 6 for the **innermost**. Color the squares by the meninges red. Color the squares by the spaces blue. Circle the one that is the location of cerebrospinal fluid.

_____ Arachnoid ❑   _____ Subarachnoid ❑   _____ Pia mater ❑

_____ Epidural ❑   _____ Dura mater ❑   _____ Subdural ❑

2. Identify the regions of the brain indicated on the following diagram. Color the somatosensory area red, the somatomotor area blue, the visual area green, and the brain stem yellow.

A. _____

B. _____

C. _____

D. _____

E. _____

F. _____

G. _____

H. _____

3. Write the name of the CNS structure that best fits each descriptive phrase.

_____ Second largest portion of the brain

_____ Includes the midbrain, pons, and medulla oblongata

_____ Includes the thalamus and hypothalamus

_____ Extends from the foramen magnum to the pons

_____ Diencephalon region regulating visceral activities

_____ Contains the apneustic and pneumotaxic centers

_____ Superior portion of the brain stem

_____ Coordinates skeletal muscles, posture, and balance

_____ Contains cardiac, vasomotor, respiratory centers

_____ Middle portion of the brainstem

4. Arrange the following numbered items in the appropriate sequence to represent the correct order of flow for cerebrospinal fluid. Write the numbers in the appropriate order on the line provided.

   1) Openings in the fourth ventricle; 2) Interventricular foramen; 3) Subarachnoid space; 4) Fourth ventricle; 5) Superior sagittal sinus; 6) Third ventricle; 7) Choroid plexus of lateral ventricle; 8) Arachnoid granulations; 9) Cerebral aqueduct

   _____ _____ _____ _____ _____ _____ _____ _____ _____

5. Identify the parts of a spinal cord and spinal nerve that are indicated by leader lines on the following diagram by writing the correct letter in the space provided before each term.

_____ Central canal   _____ Spinal nerve

_____ Dorsal horn   _____ Dorsal root ganglion

_____ Column of white matter _____ Ventral root

6. Each of the following statements about the spinal cord is false. Rewrite each statement to make it true.

   The spinal cord consists of a central core of white matter surrounded by gray matter.

Two enlargements of the spinal cord are in the thoracic and lumbar regions.

The dorsal and ventral horns contain bundles of nerve fibers, called nerve tracts.

Ascending tracts carry motor impulses to the brain.

Corticospinal tracts are ascending tracts that begin in the cerebral cortex.

Peripheral Nervous System

1. Within a nerve, each individual nerve fiber has a connective tissue covering called
_____. The nerve itself is covered by connective tissue called
_____.

2. Name the following cranial nerves.

   Three nerves that are sensory only._____

   Nerve to the muscles of facial expression._____

   Three nerves that function in eye movement._____

   Nerve that is likely to be involved if you have a
   toothache in the lower jaw. _____

   Nerve to the muscles of mastication. _____

   Nerve that allows you to nod your head. _____

3. Write the term or number that best fits each descriptive phrase.

   _____ Number of spinal nerves

   _____ Spinal nerve root that contains only sensory fibers

   _____ Complex network of nerve fibers

   _____ Number of cervical nerves

   _____ Spinal nerve root that contains only motor fibers

   _____ Nerve plexus that supplies nerves to the arm

   _____ Nerve plexus that gives rise to the phrenic nerve

   _____ Nerve plexus that gives rise to the sciatic nerve

4. Two types of efferent pathways are illustrated below. (a) Color the arrow(s) of the somatic motor pathway red and the autonomic pathway blue; (b) Identify the arrows that represent preganglionic and postganglionic fibers by writing the words in the arrow space; (c) Put an asterisk (*) by the effector that represents smooth muscle, cardiac muscle, and glands.

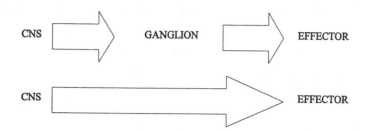

5. The following table indicates some features of the autonomic nervous system. Use a check (√) to show which division of the autonomic nervous system is involved with each feature. Both divisions may be involved in some features and both columns should be checked. S = Sympathetic division; P = Parasympathetic division.

Feature	S	P
Arises from thoracic and lumbar regions of the spinal cord		
Has terminal ganglia		
Also called the craniosacral division		
Has short preganglionic fibers		
Also called "fight-or-flight"		
Cholinergic preganglionic fibers		
Adrenergic postganglionic fibers		
Also called "rest-and-repose" system		
Dilates pupils of the eyes		
Has short postganglionic fibers		
Increases heart rate		
Cholinergic postganglionic fibers		
Dilates blood vessels to skeletal muscles		
Increases digestive enzymes		
Constricts the bronchi		

REVIEW QUESTIONS

1. What are three types of functions performed by the nervous system?

2. What are the two main divisions of the nervous system and how are these subdivided?

3. What two types of cells are found in nerve tissue?

4. What are the three basic parts of a neuron?

5. Draw a typical multipolar neuron and label the components.

6. What are the three functional types of neurons? How are they similar and how are they different?

7. What is the function of neuroglia cells? How many types are there?

8. What are the two functional characteristics of neurons?

9. What is meant by the term resting potential?

10. What happens to the neuron cell membrane when a stimulus is applied? What is an action potential?

11. How are resting conditions restored after an action potential?

12. What is meant by threshold stimulus?

13. What is a propagated action potential?

14. What is the advantage of saltatory conduction?

15. Diagram the components of a synapse and describe how an impulse is conducted from one neuron to the next.

16. What effect does an excitatory neurotransmitter have on the postsynaptic cell membrane? How does this differ from the effect of an inhibitory neurotransmitter?

17. How does a convergence circuit differ from a divergence circuit?

18. Diagram a reflex arc showing the five basic components.

19. What are the three different meninges and what is their function?

20. What are the five main regions or lobes of the cerebral hemispheres?

21. What are basal ganglia and where are they located?

22. Where are each of the following located? (a) primary sensory area; (b) primary motor area; (c) visual cortex; (d) auditory area.

23. Where is the diencephalon? What are its component parts and what are their functions?

24. What are the three parts of the brain stem and what are their functions?

25. What three vital reflex centers are located in the medulla oblongata?

26. What is the function of the cerebellum?

27. What is cerebrospinal fluid? Where is it produced? How does it circulate?

28. How does the arrangement of gray and white matter in the spinal cord differ from that in the cerebrum? What are the functions of the gray and white matter in the spinal cord?

29. What are the three connective tissue wrappings associated with a nerve?

30. What are the names of the 12 cranial nerves and what is the function of each one?

31. What is the structure and function of spinal nerves? How many are there? How are they grouped?

32. What is a nerve plexus?

33. How do the pathways in the autonomic nervous system differ from somatic efferent pathways?

34. What are the two major divisions of the autonomic nervous system? How do they differ in structure, function, and neurotransmitters?

CHAPTER QUIZ

1. Which of the following are components of the central nervous system? (a) brain and cranial nerves; (b) cranial nerves and spinal nerves; (c) spinal cord and spinal nerves; (d) brain and spinal cord; (e) sensory division and motor division.

2. Name each of the following:

   _____ Fatty covering around a neuron process

   _____ Afferent neuron process

   _____ Neuroglia cell that is phagocytic

   _____ Cell that produces myelin in the CNS

   _____ Neuron process that may have a sense receptor at its distal end

3. Number the following events in the sequence in which they occur.

   _____ Membrane becomes permeable to potassium

   _____ Threshold stimulus is applied

   _____ Sodium/potassium pump restores resting conditions

   _____ Inside of membrane is positive to the outside

   _____ Membrane becomes permeable to sodium

   _____ Membrane is polarized with potassium outside

4. Which of the following is *not* true about synaptic transmission? (a) neurotransmitters react with receptor sites on the postsynaptic membrane; (b) impulses "jump" across the synapse by saltatory conduction; (c) inhibitory neurotransmitters hyperpolarize the cell membrane; (d) excitatory neurotransmitters depolarize the cell membrane

5. Name the following:

   _____ Outermost layer of meninges

   _____ Structure that produces cerebrospinal fluid

   _____ Ventricle that is midline in the region of the diencephalon

   _____ Connective tissue covering an individual nerve fiber

   _____ Band of white fibers that connects the two cerebral hemispheres

6. Which one of the following is *not* a correctly matched pair of terms? (a) cervical plexus / phrenic nerve; (b) lumbosacral plexus / median nerve; (c) brachial plexus / radial nerve; (d) lumbosacral plexus / sciatic nerve; (e) brachial plexus / axillary nerve

7. Match each of the following with the region of the brain in which it is found.

_____ Arbor vitae

_____ Pons

_____ Insula

_____ Primary motor area

_____ Basal ganglia

_____ Thalamus

_____ Vermis

_____ Midbrain

_____ Lateral ventricles

_____ Cardiac center

A. cerebrum

B. cerebellum

C. diencephalon

D. brain stem

8. Which cranial nerve is used for each of the following?

_____ Transmits sensory impulses from an aching tooth

_____ Transmits visual impulses from the retina of the eye

_____ Transmits motor impulses to muscles for smiling

_____ Transmits motor impulses that affect heart rate

_____ Transmits motor impulses to the tongue

9. Indicate whether each of the following pertains to the (S) sympathetic, (P) parasympathetic, or (B) both divisions of the autonomic nervous system.

_____ Terminal ganglia

_____ Two neurons in the pathway

_____ Cholinergic fibers

_____ Short preganglionic fibers

_____ Adrenergic fibers

_____ Conserves energy

_____ Craniosacral division

_____ Widespread and long-lasting effect

_____ Shows little divergence

_____ Dilates blood vessels to skeletal muscles

USING CLINICAL KNOWLEDGE

1. Match the definitions on the left with the correct term from the column on the right by placing the corresponding letter in the space before the definition. Not all terms will be used.

_____	Used in the treatment of migraine headaches	A. Action potential
_____	White, fatty substance around some nerve fibers	B. ALS
_____	Antiparkinsonism agent	C. Carbidopa-levodopa
_____	Lou Gehrig's disease	D. Dihydroergotamine
_____	Nerve impulse	E. Frontal lobe
_____	Contains visual cortex	F. Medulla oblongata
_____	Painful disorder of cranial nerve V	G. Myelin
_____	Contains pneumotaxic and apneustic centers	H. Occipital lobe
		I. Pons
		J. Tic douloureux

2. Write the meaning of the following abbreviations.

_____   CVA

_____   EEG

_____   CSF

_____   ADD

_____   CT

3. Spelling is important in scientific and medical applications because only one or two incorrect letters may change the meaning. For each of the following pairs of words from this chapter, circle the one that is spelled correctly.

synapse	sinapse
ponds	pons
neurolemma	neurilemma
sclerosis	sclairosis
trigiminal	trigeminal

4. Write the meaning of the underlined portion of each word on the line preceding the word.

_____   <u>schiz</u>ophrenia

_____   epi<u>lepsy</u>

_____   <u>narc</u>olepsy

_____   an<u>alges</u>ic

_____ <u>gloss</u>opharyngeal

_____ <u>plex</u>us

_____ <u>men</u>inges

_____ an<u>esthesi</u>a

5. Use these word parts to write clinical terms that fit the given definitions.

| encephal- | hyper- | myel- | -pathy |
| -gram | -itis | neur- | -plasty |

_____ Inflammation of the brain

_____ Surgical repair of a nerve

_____ Inflammation of the spinal cord

_____ Any degenerative disease of the brain

_____ Record of a study of the spinal cord

FUN AND GAMES

First, write the words that answer the clues in the blanks of the right-hand column, one letter per blank. Then, transfer each letter to the blank with the same number in the quotation by Juvenal at the bottom of the page.

Dura mater between cerebral hemispheres $\overline{29}$ $\overline{66}$ $\overline{43}$ $\overline{0}$ $\overline{74}$ $\overline{14}$ $\overline{37}$ $\overline{70}$ $\overline{26}$ $\overline{54}$ $\overline{5}$

Type of conduction on myelinated fibers $\overline{45}$ $\overline{36}$ $\overline{21}$ $\overline{63}$ $\overline{66}$ $\overline{8}$ $\overline{33}$ $\overline{72}$ $\overline{44}$

Type of cell that produces myelin $\overline{12}$ $\overline{32}$ $\overline{7}$ $\overline{56}$ $\overline{53}$ $\overline{51}$ $\overline{18}$

"Matter" that forms columns of spinal cord $\overline{20}$ $\overline{69}$ $\overline{40}$ $\overline{39}$ $\overline{14}$

Efferent process of a neuron $\overline{23}$ $\overline{75}$ $\overline{61}$ $\overline{23}$ $\overline{37}$ $\overline{73}$ $\overline{28}$ $\overline{55}$

Posterior portion of the brain $\overline{74}$ $\overline{30}$ $\overline{54}$ $\overline{25}$ $\overline{26}$ $\overline{47}$ $\overline{3}$ $\overline{59}$ $\overline{27}$ $\overline{34}$

"Matter" formed by myelinated fibers $\overline{31}$ $\overline{7}$ $\overline{5}$ $\overline{68}$ $\overline{42}$

Extent of sympathetic effects $\overline{4}$ $\overline{50}$ $\overline{23}$ $\overline{70}$ $\overline{15}$ $\overline{65}$ $\overline{72}$ $\overline{22}$ $\overline{1}$ $\overline{23}$

Nonconducting tissue of nervous system $\overline{18}$ $\overline{70}$ $\overline{27}$ $\overline{54}$ $\overline{11}$ $\overline{24}$ $\overline{2}$ $\overline{57}$ $\overline{38}$

Junction between two neurons $\overline{6}$ $\overline{67}$ $\overline{51}$ $\overline{1}$ $\overline{46}$ $\overline{13}$ $\overline{75}$

Middle portion of the brain stem $\overline{35}$ $\overline{9}$ $\overline{61}$ $\overline{16}$

Central region of the cerebellum $\overline{41}$ $\overline{14}$ $\overline{54}$ $\overline{34}$ $\overline{60}$ $\overline{16}$

Collection of nerve cell bodies in PNS $\overline{52}$ $\overline{48}$ $\overline{18}$ $\overline{62}$ $\overline{43}$ $\overline{73}$ $\overline{64}$ $\overline{51}$

Lobe that contains visual cortex $\overline{19}$ $\overline{32}$ $\overline{74}$ $\overline{5}$ $\overline{10}$ $\overline{50}$ $\overline{8}$ $\overline{1}$ $\overline{58}$

Innermost layer of meninges $\overline{71}$ $\overline{73}$ $\overline{66}$ $\overline{34}$ $\overline{48}$ $\overline{28}$ $\overline{70}$ $\overline{37}$

Quotation:

$\overline{1}$ $\overline{2}$ $\overline{3}$ $\overline{4}$ $\overline{5}$ $\overline{6}$ $\overline{7}$ $\overline{8}$ $\overline{9}$ $\overline{10}$ $\overline{11}$ $\overline{12}$ $\overline{13}$ $\overline{14}$ $\overline{15}$ $\overline{16}$

$\overset{K}{\overline{17}}$ $\overline{18}$ $\overline{19}$ $\overline{20}$ $\overline{21}$ $\overline{22}$ $\overline{23}$ $\overline{24}$ $\overline{25}$ $\overline{26}$ $\overline{27}$ $\overline{28}$ $\overline{29}$ $\overline{30}$ $\overline{31}$,

$\overline{32}$ $\overline{33}$ $\overline{34}$ $\overline{35}$ $\overline{36}$ $\overline{37}$ $\overline{38}$ $\overline{39}$ $\overline{40}$ $\overline{41}$ $\overline{42}$ $\overline{43}$ $\overline{44}$

$\overline{45}$ $\overline{46}$ $\overline{47}$ $\overline{48}$ $\overset{K}{\overline{49}}$ $\overline{50}$ $\overline{51}$ $\overline{52}$, $\overline{53}$ $\overline{54}$ $\overline{55}$ $\overline{56}$ $\overline{57}$ $\overline{58}$ $\overline{59}$ $\overline{60}$ $\overline{61}$ $\overline{62}$

$\overline{63}$ $\overline{64}$ $\overline{65}$ $\overline{66}$ $\overline{67}$ $\overline{68}$ $\overline{69}$ $\overline{70}$ $\overline{71}$ $\overline{72}$ $\overline{73}$ $\overline{74}$ $\overline{75}$.

—Juvenal—

9

Sensory System

KEY TERMS

Accommodation
Chemoreceptor
Mechanoreceptor
Nociceptor
Photoreceptor
Proprioceptor
Sensory adaptation
Thermoreceptor

BUILDING VOCABULARY

acous-
audi-
blephar-
coch-
-cusis
dacry-
fove-
gust-
irid-
kerat-
lacr-
lith-
macul-
meat-
myring-
ocul-
olfact-
op-
ophthalm-
-opia
ot-
presby-
scler-
tympan-
vitre-
phac-

CLINICAL TERMS

Astigmatism
Audiometry
Blepharitis
Conduction deafness
Diplopia
Emmetropia
Glaucoma
Hyperopia
Labyrinthitis
Macular
Meniere's disease
Mydriasis
Myopia
Nyctalopia
Otalgia
Otomycosis
Otosclerosis
Otoscopy
Presbycusis
Presbyopia
Sensorineural deafness
Snellen chart
Tinnitus
Tonometry
Tympanitis
Vertigo

CLINICAL ABBREVIATIONS

AD
AMD

CLINICAL ABBREVIATIONS *(cont'd)*

AOM	ENT
AS	EOM
aq	ETF
BOM	ME
db	OD
DVA	OS
EENT	REM

OUTLINE/OBJECTIVES

Receptors and Sensations

- Distinguish between general senses and special senses.
  - Receptors for the general senses are widely distributed in the body.
  - Receptors for the special senses are localized.
- Classify sense receptors into five groups.
  - Receptors are classified as chemoreceptors, mechanoreceptors, nociceptors, thermoreceptors, or photoreceptors.
  - Sensory adaptation occurs when a continued stimulus decreases the sensitivity of the receptors.

General Senses

- Describe the sense receptors for touch, pressure, proprioception, temperature, and pain.
  - The receptors for touch and pressure are mechanoreceptors, which include free nerve endings, Meissner's corpuscles, and Pacinian corpuscles.
  - Proprioception is the sense of position or orientation. The receptors are mechanoreceptors including Golgi tendon organs and muscle spindles.
  - Temperature changes are detected by thermoreceptors, which are free nerve endings. Some are sensitive to heat, others to cold, and temperature extremes also stimulate pain receptors.
  - Receptors for pain are called nociceptors, which are free nerve endings that are stimulated by tissue damage.

Gustatory Sense

- Locate the four different taste sensations and follow the impulse pathway from stimulus to the cerebral cortex.
  - Receptors for taste are chemoreceptors located in the taste buds.
  - Taste buds, the organs for taste, are located on the walls of the papillae that are on the surface of the tongue.
  - Taste buds contain the taste cells and supporting cells. Taste hairs on the taste cells function as the receptors.
  - Sweet, salty, sour, and bitter are the four taste sensations. Sweet is located at the tip of the tongue, salty is on the anterior sides of the tongue, sour is on the posterior sides of the tongue, and bitter is at the back of the tongue.
  - Impulses for taste are transmitted along the facial nerve or the glossopharyngeal nerve to the sensory cortex of the parietal lobe.

Olfactory Sense

- Locate the sense receptors for smell and trace the impulse pathway to the cerebral cortex.
  — The sense of smell is called olfaction.
  — The receptors for the sense of smell are chemoreceptors and are located in the olfactory epithelium of the nasal cavity.
  — The olfactory neurons enter the olfactory bulb. Impulses are transmitted along the olfactory tracts to the olfactory cortex in the temporal lobe.
  — The senses of taste and smell are closely related and complement each other.

Visual Sense

- Describe the structure of the eye and the significance of each component.
  — Protective features of the eye include the bony orbit, the eyebrows, eyelids, and eyelashes, which help to protect the eye from foreign particles and irritants, and the lacrimal apparatus, which produces tears that moisten and cleanse the eye. Tears contain an enzyme that helps destroy bacteria.
  — The sclera and cornea are parts of the outermost layer, or fibrous tunic, of the eye. They give shape to the eye, and the cornea refracts light rays.
  — The middle, or vascular, tunic includes the choroid, ciliary body, and iris. The choroid absorbs excess light rays; the ciliary body changes the shape of the lens; and the iris regulates the size of the pupil.
  — The retina is the innermost layer, or nervous tunic, of the eye. It contains the receptor cells.
  — The lens, suspensory ligaments, and ciliary body form a partition that divides the interior of the eye into two cavities. The anterior cavity is filled with aqueous humor and the posterior cavity is filled with vitreous humor. Both the aqueous and vitreous humors refract light rays.
- Explain how light focuses on the retina.
  — Refraction is the bending of light rays as they travel between substances of differing optical densities. The refractive media in the eye are the cornea, aqueous humor, lens, and vitreous humor.
  — In the normal relaxed eye, the four refractive media sufficiently bend the light rays from objects at least 20 feet away to focus on the retina.
  — When the eyes accommodate for close vision, the ciliary muscle contracts, the suspensory ligaments become less taut, and the lens becomes more convex so light rays have sufficient refraction to focus on the retina.
- Identify the photoreceptor cells in the retina, describe the mechanism by which nerve impulses are triggered in response to light, and trace the impulse to the visual cortex.
  — Rods are the photoreceptors for black and white vision and for vision in dim light. Cones are the receptors for color vision and visual acuity. The rods and cones are located in the retina.
  — Rods contain rhodopsin, which breaks down into opsin and retinal when it is exposed to light. This reaction triggers a nerve impulse.
  — Cones, concentrated in the fovea centralis, function in a manner similar to rods. Color is possible because one type of cone is sensitive to green light, one is sensitive to blue light, and the third responds to red light.
  — Visual impulses triggered by the rods and cones travel on the optic nerve to the optic chiasma. From the optic chiasma, the impulses travel on the optic tracts to the thalamus. From there, the impulses travel on optic radiations to the visual cortex in the occipital lobe.

Auditory Sense

- Describe the structure of the ear and the contribution each region makes to the sense of hearing.

— The outer, or external, ear, which includes the auricle and external auditory meatus, ends at the tympanic membrane. The auricle collects the sound waves and directs them toward the external auditory meatus, which serves as a passageway to the tympanic membrane.

— The middle ear contains three tiny bones called auditory ossicles, the malleus, incus, and stapes. The auditory ossicles transmit sound vibrations from the tympanic membrane to the oval window.

— The inner ear consists of a bony labyrinth that surrounds a membranous labyrinth. It includes the vestibule, semicircular canals, and cochlea. The cochlea is the part that functions in hearing. The membranous labyrinth of the cochlea is the cochlear duct, which contains endolymph. The organ of Corti, located on the basilar membrane in the cochlear duct, contains the receptors for sound.

- Summarize the sequence of events in the initiation of auditory impulses and trace these impulses to the auditory cortex.

— Sound waves cause vibration of the tympanic membrane. Auditory ossicles transmit the vibrations through the middle ear to the oval window.

— Movement of the oval window passes the vibrations to the perilymph in the scala vestibuli and scala tympani in the inner ear. This creates corresponding oscillations in the vestibular and basilar membranes of the cochlear duct.

— As the basilar membrane moves up and down, the hairs on the hair cells of the organ of Corti rub against the tectorial membrane. Mechanical deformation of the hairs triggers the nerve impulses.

— The interpretation of pitch is mediated by the portion of the basilar membrane that vibrates, and loudness is interpreted by the number of hair cells that are stimulated.

— Cranial nerve VIII transmits auditory impulses to the medulla oblongata. From there, the impulses travel to the thalamus, and then to the auditory cortex of the temporal lobe.

Sense of Equilibrium

- Identify and describe the structure of the components of the ear involved in static equilibrium and those involved in dynamic equilibrium.

— Static equilibrium occurs when the head is motionless. It is involved in evaluating the position of the head relative to gravity. The organ of static equilibrium is the macula, located within the utricle and saccule, which are portions of the membranous labyrinth inside the vestibule.

— Dynamic equilibrium is the equilibrium of motion and occurs when the head is moving. The receptors for dynamic equilibrium are located in the crista ampullaris within the ampullae at the base of the semicircular canals.

- Summarize the events in the initiation of impulses for static equilibrium and for dynamic equilibrium, and identify the cranial nerve that transmits these impulses to the cerebral cortex.

— For both static and dynamic equilibrium, as the head moves, hairs on the receptor cells bend and trigger an impulse, which is transmitted to the central nervous system on cranial nerve VIII.

LEARNING EXERCISES

Receptors and Sensations

1. Senses with receptors that are widely distributed within the body are called _____ senses. If the receptors are localized in a specific region, they are called _____ senses.

2. In the blank at the left, write the type of sense receptor that responds to the indicated stimulus.

_____ Light energy

_____ Changes in pressure or movement

_____ Temperature changes

_____ Tissue damage

_____ Changes in chemical composition

3. _____ occurs when certain receptors are continually stimulated and no longer respond unless the stimulus becomes more intense.

General Senses

1. Place a check (√) in the space before each correct association.

_____ Pacinian corpuscles / mechanoreceptors

_____ Pain / nociceptors

_____ Mechanoreceptors / proprioception

_____ Golgi tendon organs / touch

_____ Meissner's corpuscles / heavy pressure

2. Circle the word in the parentheses that makes the statement true.

(Thermoreceptors / Nociceptors) exhibit rapid sensory adaptation.

(Proprioceptors / Nociceptors) may send impulses after the stimulus is removed.

Gustatory Sense

1. Write the terms that best fit the following descriptive phrases.

_____ Another name for sense of taste

_____ Projections on tongue that contain taste buds

_____ Structures that project through a taste pore

_____ Type of receptors involved in taste

2. Write the terms that best fit the following descriptive phrases about taste.

_____ Four types of taste sensations

_____ Transmits impulses from anterior tongue

_____ Transmits impulses from posterior tongue

_____ Location of sensory cortex for taste in brain

Olfactory Sense

1. The chemoreceptors for olfaction are found in the olfactory epithelium located in the _____.

2. The olfactory nerve, cranial nerve number _____, transmits impulses to the olfactory cortex in the _____ lobe of the brain.

3. Airborne molecules may stimulate the sense of _____ and the sense of _____ at the same time.

Visual Sense

1. Write the terms that best fit the following descriptive phrases about the eye.

_____ Gland that produces tears

_____ Mucous membrane that lines the eyelid

_____ White part of the fibrous tunic

_____ Anterior transparent part of the fibrous tunic

_____ Pigmented vascular tunic

_____ Opening in the center of the iris

_____ Fluid in the anterior cavity of the eye

_____ Muscles that regulate size of the pupil

_____ Muscles that control shape of the lens

_____ Function of ciliary processes

_____ Nervous tunic of the eye

_____ Photoreceptor cells

_____ Region where the optic nerve penetrates the eye

_____ Depression in center of the macula lutea

_____ Gel-like fluid in the posterior cavity

2. In the normal eye, light rays from distant objects are bent so they focus on the retina. This bending of light rays is called _____.

3. Circle the correct word in each pair to make true statements. Accommodation is the adjustment needed to focus light rays for (distant/close) vision. To focus light rays from close objects, the ciliary muscle (relaxes/contracts), which (increases/decreases) the tension on the suspensory ligaments. When this happens, the lens becomes (thicker/thinner) and light rays are bent (more/less). In addition, the pupil (dilates/constricts).

4. Identify the listed structures of the bulbus oculi by matching them with the correct letters from the diagram. Color the two surfaces and two liquid media that bend light rays.

_____ Anterior cavity

_____ Choroid

_____ Ciliary body

_____ Cornea

_____ Eyelid

_____ Iris

_____ Lens

_____ Optic nerve

_____ Posterior cavity

_____ Retina

_____ Sclera

_____ Suspensory ligaments

5. Write the terms that best fit the following descriptive phrases about photoreceptors.

_____ Receptors for bright light vision

_____ Pigment contained in rods

_____ Receptors for color vision

_____ Colors of light absorbed by color receptors

_____ Receptors for dim light vision

_____ Pigment that is very light-sensitive

_____ Receptors not present in the fovea

_____ Vitamin required for photopigment synthesis

_____ Area of retina lacking photoreceptors

_____ Photoreceptors that exhibit greater convergence

6. Use the numbers 1 through 7 in the blanks to indicate the order of impulse transmission in the visual pathway. Use number 1 for the origination of the impulse and number 7 for the final visual cortex.

_____ Optic chiasma   _____ Optic tract   _____ Photoreceptors

_____ Optic nerve   _____ Thalamus   _____ Optic radiations

_____ Occipital lobe

Auditory Sense

1. Identify the listed structures of the ear by matching them with the correct letters from the diagram. Use red to color the external ear, yellow for the middle ear, and blue for the inner ear.

_____   Ampulla

_____   Auditory tube

_____   Auricle

_____   Cochlea

_____   External auditory canal

_____   Incus

_____   Malleus

_____   Semicircular canals

_____   Stapes

_____   Tympanic membrane

_____   Vestibule

_____   Vestibulocochlear nerve

2. Write the terms that best fit the following descriptive phrases about the inner ear.

_____   Series of interconnecting chambers in temporal bone

_____   Membranous tubes inside bony labyrinth

_____   Fluid inside the membranous labyrinth

_____   Fluid outside the membranous labyrinth

_____   Coiled portion of bony labyrinth

_____   Coiled portion of membranous labyrinth

_____   Membrane upon which the organ of Corti rests

_____   Membrane between scala vestibuli and cochlear duct

_____   Membrane between scala tympani and cochlear duct

3. Complete the following sentences about the events in the initiation of auditory impulses by writing the correct words in the spaces on the left.

1. _____

2. _____

3. _____

4. _____

5. _____

6. _____

7. _____

8. _____

9. _____

10. _____

Sound waves travel through the external auditory meatus until they reach the <u>1</u>, which starts to vibrate. These vibrations are transferred to the <u>2</u>, then the <u>3</u>, then the <u>4</u>, which is attached to the oval window. The oval window passes the vibrations to the <u>5</u> in the scala vestibuli of the inner ear. As vibrations pass through the scala vestibuli, they create corresponding movement of the <u>6</u> within the scala media. Finally, the vibrations are transferred to the basilar membrane and as it moves up and down, the <u>7</u> of the organ of Corti rub against the <u>8</u> and bend. This mechanical deformation initiates the nerve impulses that result in hearing. Pitch is determined by the region of the <u>9</u> that vibrates in response to the sound. Loudness is determined by magnitude of <u>10</u> of the membrane.

Sense of Equilibrium

1. Write the terms that best fit the following descriptive phrases about the sense of equilibrium.

_____ Equilibrium of rotational or angular movement

_____ Position of head relative to gravity

_____ Receptor organ for static equilibrium

_____ Chambers containing static equilibrium organs (2)

_____

_____ Calcium carbonate crystals on surface of the macula

_____ Receptor organ for dynamic equilibrium

_____ Location of dynamic equilibrium receptor organ

REVIEW QUESTIONS

1. What is the difference in the distribution of the receptors for the general senses and the special senses?

2. What are the five classes of sense receptors?

3. What is meant by sensory adaptation?

4. Name three receptors involved in the sense of touch and pressure.

5. What term is given to the sense of position or orientation? Name two receptors involved with this sense.

6. What stimulates nociceptors?

7. Where are the receptors for taste located?

8. Name the four different types of taste and map the location of their receptors on the surface of the tongue.

9. What cranial nerve is involved in the sense of smell?

10. In what ways are the senses of taste and smell related?

11. What bones are in the orbit of the eye?

12. What is the function of eyelashes, eyelids, and eyebrows?

13. Where are tears produced and what is their function?

14. Draw and label a diagram that illustrates the three layers of the bulbus oculi.

15. Where are the aqueous humor and vitreous humor located?

16. What parts of the bulbus oculi bend light rays so they focus on the retina?

17. How does the ciliary body act to change the shape of the lens for accommodation?

18. What are the rods and cones and where are they located?

19. How do photoreceptor cells trigger nerve impulses?

20. Which cranial nerve transmits visual impulses and where are these impulses interpreted?

21. Label a diagram of the ear.

22. What three bones are found in the ear?

23. What fluid is found inside the bony labyrinth but outside the membranous labyrinth?

24. In what specific portion of the ear are the auditory receptors located?

25. How are sound vibrations converted into auditory impulses?

26. How does the ear distinguish between loud sounds and soft or quiet sounds?

27. In what part of the brain is the auditory cortex located?

28. What is the difference between static equilibrium and dynamic equilibrium?

29. Where are the receptors for static equilibrium located?

30. Where are the receptors for dynamic equilibrium located?

31. What mechanical event triggers impulses for equilibrium?

32. Which cranial nerve transmits impulses for equilibrium to the central nervous system?

CHAPTER QUIZ

1. Each of the following sensations is preceded by two blanks. In the first blank, indicate whether the sensation is one of the general senses or one of the special senses. In the second blank, indicate the type of receptor involved. Use the letter key that is given.

____ ____	Vision	G = general sense	
____ ____	Touch	S = special sense	
____ ____	Taste		
____ ____	Smell		
____ ____	Cold shower	C = chemoreceptor	
____ ____	Toothache	M = mechanoreceptor	
____ ____	Static equilibrium	N = nociceptor	
____ ____	Pressure	P = photoreceptor	
____ ____	Pain from a burn	T = thermoreceptor	
____ ____	Hearing		

2. Which of the following is *not* true about the sense of taste? (a) it is also called the gustatory sense; (b) in order to be tasted, substances must be dissolved; (c) receptors for the different tastes are randomly distributed over the surface of the tongue; (d) the facial and glossopharyngeal nerves transmit impulses for taste to the parietal lobe; (e) the receptors for taste are located in the taste buds.

3. Which of the following is *not* true about protective features of the eye? (a) the frontal, ethmoid, and zygomatic bones contribute to the bony socket for the eye; (b) the gland that produces tears is located along the upper medial margin of the eye; (c) tears contain an enzyme that helps destroy pathogenic bacteria; (d) the eyes are opened by contraction of the levator palpebrae superioris muscle; (e) sebaceous glands are associated with the eyelashes.

4. Which of the following represents the correct sequence for the visual pathway?
   (a) optic tract, optic chiasma, optic nerve, thalamus, optic radiations, visual cortex;
   (b) optic radiations, optic tract, optic chiasma, optic nerve, thalamus, visual cortex;
   (c) optic nerve, thalamus, optic tract, optic chiasma, optic radiations, visual cortex;
   (d) optic nerve, optic chiasma, optic tract, thalamus, optic radiations, visual cortex;
   (e) optic tract, thalamus, optic nerve, optic chiasma, optic radiations, visual cortex;

5. Name the following:

   _____ Innermost tunic of the eyeball

   _____ White portion of the outer tunic

   _____ Fluid in the anterior cavity of the eye

   _____ Muscle that contracts to make the lens more convex

   _____ Center depression in the macula lutea

_____ Receptors for color vision

_____ Contains muscles that change the size of the pupil

_____ Region where the optic nerve penetrates the eye

_____ First structure that refracts light entering the eye

_____ Pigment in the rods

6. Indicate whether each of the following parts of the ear is involved in hearing (H), equilibrium (E), or both (B).

_____ Malleus, incus, stapes

_____ Membranous labyrinth

_____ Semicircular canals

_____ Cochlea

_____ Utricle and saccule

_____ Tectorial membrane

_____ Endolymph

_____ Hair cells

_____ Organ of Corti

_____ Vestibulocochlear nerve

7. Name the following organs located in the ear:

_____ Contains the receptor cells for hearing

_____ Contains the receptor cells for static equilibrium

_____ Contains the receptor cells for dynamic equilibrium

USING CLINICAL KNOWLEDGE

1. Match the definitions on the left with the correct term from the column on the right by placing the corresponding letter in the space before the definition. Not all terms will be used.

_____	Cause pupil dilation	A. Astigmatism
_____	Responds to tissue damage	B. Cycloplegic agents
_____	Inflammation of the inner ear	C. Emmetropia
_____	Impairment of hearing due to aging	D. Glaucoma
_____	Paralyze ciliary muscle to prevent accommodation	E. Labyrinthitis
_____	Fungal infection of the external ear	F. Meniere's disease
_____	Night blindness	G. Mydriatic agents
_____	Ringing or buzzing sound in the ears	H. Nociceptors
_____	Defective curvature of the cornea	I. Nyctalopia
_____	Characterized by increased intraocular pressure	J. Otalgia
		K. Otomycosis
		L. Otosclerosis
		M. Presbycusis
		N. Tinnitis

2. Write the meaning of the following abbreviations.

_____ REM

_____ EOM

_____ EENT

_____ OS

_____ AD

3. Spelling is important in scientific and medical applications because only one or two incorrect letters may change the meaning. All of the following words are from this chapter and three are spelled incorrectly. Place a √ in the space preceding the words that are spelled correctly and write the correct spelling in the space preceding the misspelled words.

_____ eustachian

_____ oldfactory

_____ gustatary

_____ lacrimal

_____ retna

4. Write the meaning of the underlined portion of each word on the line preceding the word.

_____ blepharitis

_____ hyperopia

_____ phacoemulsification

_____ myringitis

_____ dacryolith

5. Use these word parts to write clinical terms that fit the given definitions.

dacry-   irid-   myring-   oto-   -plasty
-ectomy   kerat-   -oma   -otomy

_____ Excision of a full-thickness piece of the iris

_____ Incision of the cornea

_____ Plastic surgery of the external ear

_____ Excision of the tympanic membrane

_____ Tumorlike swelling due to obstruction of the lacrimal
                                 duct

FUN AND GAMES

Braille is a system of writing for the blind that uses characters made up of raised dots. Each letter of the alphabet is represented by a specific pattern of dots as indicated in the alphabet that is given below. By learning this alphabet, the blind person can read with his or her fingers by feeling the patterns of raised dots.

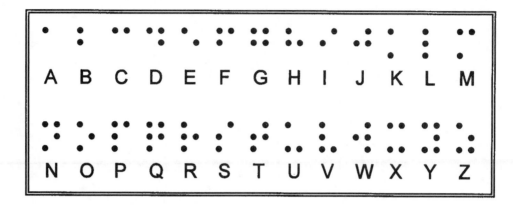

Use the Braille alphabet given above to decipher this quotation by Ralph Waldo Emerson that reflects on the versatility of the eyes.

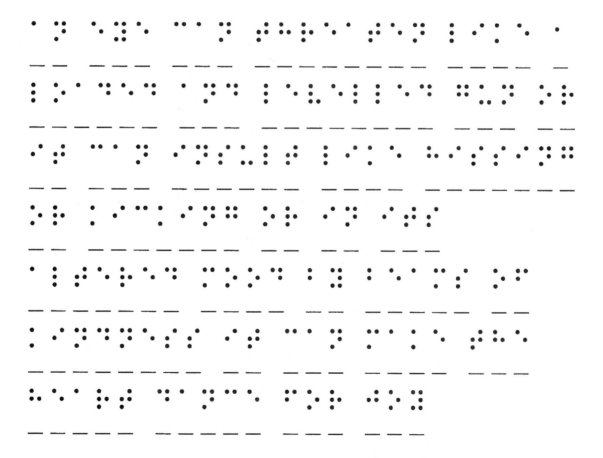

10

Endocrine System

KEY TERMS

Adenohypophysis
Endocrine gland
Exocrine gland
Hormone
Negative feedback
Neurohypophysis
Prostaglandins
Target tissue

BUILDING VOCABULARY

-ac
acr-
ad-
aden-
-agon
-amine
andr-
calc-
cortic-
crin-
di-
dips-
-gen-
-gest-
glyc-
gonad-
lact-
-megaly
oxy-
para-
-physis
pin-
-ren-
ster-

test-
-toc-
trop-
-uria

CLINICAL TERMS

Acromegaly
Adenoma
Anabolic steroids
Cretinism
Cushing's syndrome
Diabetes insipidus
Diabetes mellitus
Endocrinology
Endocrinopathy
Exophthalmic
Glucose tolerance test
Myxedema
Polydipsia
Polyphagia
Polyuria
Progeria

CLINICAL ABBREVIATIONS

ACTH
ADH
CS
DKA
DR
FSH
GDM
GH
HCG
ICSH

CLINICAL ABBREVIATIONS *(cont'd)*

IDDM	PRL
LH	PTH
MSH	T_3
NIDDM	T_4
OXT	

OUTLINE/OBJECTIVES

Introduction to the Endocrine System

- Compare the actions of the nervous system and the endocrine system.
  - The nervous system acts through electrical impulses and neurotransmitters; the effect is localized and of short duration.
  - The endocrine system acts through chemicals called hormones; the effect is generalized and of long-term duration.

Characteristics of Hormones

- Compare the major chemical classes of hormones.
  - Hormones are classified chemically as either proteins or steroids.
  - Most hormones in the body are proteins or protein derivatives. The receptors for these hormones are located on the cell membrane.
  - The sex hormones and those from the adrenal cortex are steroids. The receptors for these hormones are located within the cytoplasm of the cell.
- Discuss the general mechanisms of hormone action.
  - Hormones react with receptor sites on selected cells. The cells that have receptor sites for a specific hormone make up the target tissue for that hormone.
  - Protein hormones react with receptors on the surface of the cell; steroids react with receptors inside the cell.
  - Many hormones are regulated by a negative feedback mechanism; some hormones are secreted in response to other hormones; and a third method for regulating hormone secretion is by direct nerve stimulation.

Endocrine Glands and Their Hormones

- Identify the major endocrine glands and discuss their hormones and functions: pituitary, thyroid, parathyroid, adrenal, pancreas, gonads, thymus, and pineal.
  - The pituitary gland is divided into an anterior lobe, or adenohypophysis, which is regulated by releasing hormones from the hypothalamus, and a posterior lobe, or neurohypophysis, which is regulated by nerve stimulation.
  - Hormones of the anterior lobe (adenohypophysis) include the following:
    - Growth hormone (GH), or somatotropic hormone (STH), promotes protein synthesis, which results in growth.
    - Thyroid stimulating hormone (TSH) stimulates the activity of the follicular cells of the thyroid gland.
    - Adrenocorticotropic hormone (ACTH) stimulates activity of the adrenal cortex, particularly the secretion of cortisol.

- Follicle stimulating hormone (FSH) is a gonadotropin that stimulates the development of ova in the ovaries and sperm in the testes. It also stimulates the production of estrogen in the female.
- Luteinizing hormone (LH), another gonadotropin, causes ovulation and the secretion of progesterone and estrogen in the female. In the male it stimulates the production of testosterone.
- Prolactin promotes the development of glandular tissue in the breast and stimulates the production of milk.

— Hormones of the posterior lobe (neurohypophysis) include the following:
- Antidiuretic hormone (ADH) promotes reabsorption of water in the kidney tubules.
- Oxytocin causes uterine muscle contraction and ejection of milk from the lactating breast.

— Thyroid gland hormones include thyroxine, triiodothyronine, and calcitonin.
- Both thyroxine and triiodothyronine require iodine for synthesis. About 95% of active thyroid hormone is thyroxine. Thyroid hormone secretion is regulated by a negative feedback mechanism that involves the amount of circulating hormone, the hypothalamus, and TSH from the adenohypophysis. Thyroid hormones affect the metabolism of carbohydrates, proteins, and lipids. Hyperthyroidism is characterized by a high metabolic rate. Hypothyroidism leads to conditions related to decreased metabolism.
- Calcitonin is produced by parafollicular cells in the thyroid gland. It reduces calcium levels in the blood.

— Parathyroid glands are embedded on the posterior surface of the thyroid gland. Parathyroid hormone, antagonistic to calcitonin, increases blood calcium levels. Hypoparathyroidism reduces blood calcium levels, which may result in nerve irritability. Hyperparathyroidism results in calcium loss from bones and precipitation in abnormal places.

— The adrenal (suprarenal) gland is separated into a cortex and a medulla.
- All hormones from the adrenal cortex are steroids and are regulated by a negative feedback mechanism involving the hypothalamus and ACTH from the adenohypophysis. Hormones from the adrenal cortex are classified as either mineralocorticoids, glucocorticoids, or sex steroids. The principal mineralocorticoid is aldosterone, which promotes sodium ion reabsorption in the kidney tubules. The principal glucocorticoid is cortisol, which increases blood glucose levels and helps to counteract the inflammatory response. Sex steroids from the adrenal cortex have minimal effect compared to the hormones from the ovaries and testes.
- The two hormones produced by the adrenal medulla are epinephrine and norepinephrine. About 80% of the product is epinephrine. Epinephrine and norepinephrine prepare the body for strenuous activity and stress. The effect of epinephrine and norepinephrine is similar to that of the sympathetic nervous system but lasts up to ten times longer.

— The endocrine portion of the pancreas consists of the pancreatic islets, or islets of Langerhans. Alpha cells in the islets produce glucagon and the beta cells produce insulin. The principal action of glucagon is to raise blood glucose levels. Insulin, antagonistic to glucagon, decreases blood glucose levels.

— Testes produce the male sex hormones, which are collectively called androgens. The principal androgen is testosterone, which is responsible for the development and maintenance of male secondary sex characteristics.

— The ovaries produce estrogen and progesterone. Estrogen is responsible for the development and maintenance of female secondary sex characteristics. Progesterone maintains the uterine lining for pregnancy.

— The pineal gland extends posteriorly from the third ventricle of the brain. Secretory cells, called pinealocytes, synthesize and secrete the hormone melatonin. This hormone inhibits gonadotropin releasing hormone from the hypothalamus, which inhibits reproductive functions. Melatonin also regulates circadian rhythms.

— The thymus, located near the midline in the anterior portion of the thoracic cavity, produces the hormone thymosin. Thymosin plays an important role in the development of the immune system of the body.

• Name and describe the function of at least one hormone from the (a) gastric mucosa; (b) small intestine; (c) heart; and (d) placenta.

— The gastric mucosa, the lining of the stomach, produces gastrin, a hormone that stimulates the production of hydrochloric acid and the enzyme pepsin.

— Cells in the duodenum of the small intestine secrete cholecystokinin and secretin. Cholecystokinin stimulates contraction of the gallbladder and stimulates the pancreas to produce an enzyme-rich fluid. Secretin stimulates the pancreas to produce a fluid that is rich in bicarbonate ions.

— Special cells in the wall of the heart produce atrial natriuretic hormone. The primary effect of this hormone is the loss of sodium and water in the urine, which decreases blood volume and blood pressure.

— The placenta is a temporary endocrine gland that secretes human chorionic gonadotropin (HCG), which maintains the uterine lining during the first part of pregnancy.

Prostaglandins

• Differentiate between hormones and prostaglandins.

— Prostaglandins are hormone-like molecules that are derived from arachidonic acid.

— They are produced by cells widely distributed throughout the body; their effect is localized near their origin; and their effect is immediate and short-term.

— Prostaglandins are not stored; they are synthesized when needed.

LEARNING EXERCISES

Introduction to the Endocrine System

1. For each of the following phrases, place an N in the space provided if the phrase pertains to the nervous system and an E if it pertains to the endocrine system.

    _____   Acts through hormones

    _____   Effect is localized

    _____   Acts through electrical impulses

    _____   Effect is of short-term duration

    _____   Effect is generalized and long-term

2. Exocrine glands have _____ that carry the secretory product to a surface. In contrast, _____ are ductless and secrete their product directly into the _____ for transport to the target tissue.

Characteristics of Hormones

1. Write the terms that best fit the following descriptive phrases about the characteristics of hormones.

_____   Chemical nature of nonsteroid hormones

_____   Hormones that are lipid derivatives

_____   Cells that have hormone receptors

_____   Location of receptors for protein hormones

_____   Location of receptors for steroid hormones

_____   Mechanisms for controlling secretion (3)

_____

_____

2. Complete the following sentences about the reaction of a hormone with its receptor.

1. _____

2. _____

3. _____

4. _____

5. _____

6. _____

7. _____

8. _____

9. _____

10. _____

A 1 hormone combines with a receptor on the surface of the cell. This activates an enzyme within the membrane, called 2, and the enzyme diffuses into the cytoplasm where it catalyzes the production of 3. This substance, a derivative of 4, activates other enzymes that alter cellular activity. The 5 is called the first messenger and 6 is called the second messenger. A 7 hormone diffuses through the cell membrane and reacts with a 8 within the cytoplasm. The complex that forms enters the 9 and reacts with 10 to stimulate protein synthesis.

Endocrine Glands and Their Hormones

1. Identify the listed endocrine glands by matching them with the correct letters from the diagram.

   _____ Adrenal gland

   _____ Ovaries

   _____ Pancreas

   _____ Parathyroid

   _____ Pineal gland

   _____ Pituitary gland

   _____ Thymus

   _____ Thyroid

   _____ Testes

2. Match each of the following phrases with the region of the pituitary gland that it describes.

   _____ Secretes ADH   A = adenohypophysis

   _____ Stimulated by releasing hormones   B = neurohypophysis

   _____ Secretes prolactin

   _____ Derived from nervous tissue

   _____ Secretes oxytocin

   _____ Derived from embryonic oral cavity

   _____ Secretes TSH

   _____ Secretes growth hormone

   _____ Secretes ACTH

   _____ Regulated by nerve stimulation

3. Write the name of the pituitary hormones that best match the following functions.

   _____ Stimulates secretion of thyroid hormone

   _____ Stimulates the adrenal cortex

   _____ Stimulates ovulation

   _____ Stimulates uterine contractions

   _____ Increases water reabsorption

_____ Stimulates spermatogenesis

_____ Stimulates protein synthesis and growth

_____ Stimulates ejection of milk

_____ Stimulates production of testosterone

_____ Stimulates milk production

4. Match each of the following phrases with the correct hormone from the thyroid and parathyroid glands.

_____ Secreted by parafollicular cells   C = calcitonin

_____ Requires iodine for production   P = parathyroid hormone

_____ Increases blood calcium levels   T = thyroxine

_____ Secreted by thyroid follicles

_____ Increases rate of metabolism

_____ Reduces blood calcium levels

_____ Increases osteoclast activity

_____ Hyposecretion leads to nerve excitability

5. Write the terms that best fit the following descriptive phrases about the adrenal gland.

_____ Region regulated by nerve impulses

_____ Group of hormones from the outer cortical layer

_____ Primary mineralocorticoid hormone

_____ Region regulated by negative feedback

_____ Primary glucocorticoid

_____ Increases blood sodium levels

_____ Counteracts inflammatory response

_____ Secreted by the innermost layer of the cortex

_____ Hormones from the adrenal medulla (2)

_____

6. Indicate whether each descriptive phrase refers to insulin or to glucagon by writing the appropriate word in the space provided.

_____ Secreted in response to elevated blood glucose levels

_____ Secreted by the alpha cells

_____ Promotes breakdown of glycogen into glucose

_____ Secreted by the beta cells

_____ Stimulates liver to store glucose as glycogen

_____ Secreted in response to low blood glucose levels

_____ Increases blood glucose levels

_____ Decreases blood glucose levels

_____ Hyposecretion may result in diabetes mellitus

7. Each of the following hormones is preceded by two blanks. In the first blank, indicate the source of the hormone, and in the second blank, indicate a function of the hormone from the lists provided.

_____ _____	Testosterone	A. heart	1. alkaline fluid from pancreas
_____ _____	Melatonin	B. ovaries	2. contraction of gallbladder
_____ _____	Thymosin	C. pineal gland	3. decreases blood volume
_____ _____	Estrogen	D. placenta	4. development of lymphocytes
_____ _____	HCG	E. small intestine	5. female sex characteristics
_____ _____	Gastrin	F. stomach	6. maintains pregnancy
_____ _____	Secretin	G. testes	7. male sex characteristics
_____ _____	Progesterone	H. thymus	8. prepares uterus for pregnancy
_____ _____	Cholecystokinin		9. production of HCl in stomach
_____ _____	Atrial peptin		10. regulation of body rhythms

Prostaglandins

1. Prostaglandins are similar to hormones, but they are different in many ways. They are derivatives of _____, and the cells that produce them are _____ throughout the body.

2. In contrast to hormones, the effects of prostaglandins are _____, _____, and _____.

REVIEW QUESTIONS

1. How does the endocrine system compare with the nervous system in its regulatory function?

2. How do endocrine glands differ from exocrine glands in their mode of secretion?

3. What are the two principal chemical classes of hormones?

4. How do hormones recognize their target tissues?

5. Where are the receptor sites for protein hormones located? Where are the receptor sites for steroid hormones located?

6. List three different mechanisms for regulating hormone secretion.

7. How does a negative feedback system function to regulate hormone secretion?

8. List the eight major endocrine glands.

9. How is the secretory activity of the adenohypophysis controlled? Neurohypophysis?

10. List six hormones secreted by the adenohypophysis.

11. For each of the six hormones secreted by the adenohypophysis, write a sentence that describes its action.

12. What gland secretes antidiuretic hormone and oxytocin? What is the function of these two hormones?

13. What portion of the thyroid gland secretes the hormones that contain iodine?

14. What causes a simple goiter?

15. What are the effects of hypersecretion and hyposecretion of thyroxine?

16. What is the function of calcitonin and where is it produced?

17. Where are the parathyroid glands located and what is the function of the hormone they produce?

18. How do calcitonin and parathyroid hormone differ in function?

19. How do the adrenal cortex and medulla differ in the way their secretory activity is regulated?

20. What hormones are produced by the adrenal cortex? What are their functions?

21. Which adrenocortical hormones are vital to life and why?

22. What hormones have an effect that is similar to that of the sympathetic nervous system?

23. What constitutes the endocrine portion of the pancreas?

24. What cells produce glucagon? Insulin?

25. What is the difference in action between glucagon and insulin?

26. What is the main source of testosterone?

27. What two hormones are produced by the ovaries?

28. What two functions are attributed to melatonin?

29. Of what importance is the thymus gland?

30. How do prostaglandins differ from hormones?

31. What are some of the functions of prostaglandins?

CHAPTER QUIZ

1. Classify the following hormones as either protein (P) or steroid (S) in chemical composition.

   _____ Growth hormone   _____ Insulin

   _____ Epinephrine   _____ Cortisol

   _____ Aldosterone   _____ Follicle-stimulating hormone

2. Use the term "receptor sites" to write a sentence that defines target tissue.

3. Match each of the following hormones with the primary gland that secretes it.

   A. adenohypophysis   G. pancreas, beta cells
   B. adrenal cortex   H. parathyroid
   C. adrenal medulla   I. pineal
   D. neurohypophysis   J. testes
   E. ovaries   K. thymus
   F. pancreas, alpha cells   L. thyroid

   _____ Growth hormone   _____ Calcitonin

   _____ Gonadotropins   _____ Antidiuretic hormone

   _____ Epinephrine   _____ Cortisol

   _____ Melatonin   _____ Glucagon

   _____ Luteinizing hormone   _____ Testosterone

   _____ Oxytocin   _____ Thyroxine

   _____ Aldosterone   _____ TSH

   _____ Prolactin   _____ Thymosin

   _____ Progesterone   _____ Estrogen

   _____ Insulin   _____ ACTH

4. Name the hormone that is responsible for each of the following effects.

   _____ Promotes the development of sperm

   _____ Stimulates the production of milk

   _____ Plays a role in the development of immunity

   _____ Affects the body's rate of metabolism

   _____ Promotes the production of progesterone

   _____ Increases blood calcium levels

   _____ Regulates circadian rhythms

_____   Causes uterine contractions

_____   Promotes production of estrogen

_____   Decreases blood glucose levels

_____   Promotes kidney reabsorption of sodium ions

_____   Responds in stress or emergency situations

_____   Has an anti-inflammatory effect

_____   Promotes the production of testosterone

_____   Decreases blood calcium levels

5. For each of the following statements, indicate whether the statement pertains to prostaglandins (P) or hormones (H).

_____   Derived from arachidonic acid

_____   Transported to distant sites in the blood

_____   May be stored in the body

_____   Produced by cells widely distributed in the body

_____   Have a localized effect

_____   Derived from proteins and lipids

USING CLINICAL KNOWLEDGE

1. Match the definitions on the left with the correct term from the column on the right by placing the corresponding letter in the space before the definition. Not all terms will be used.

_____ Synthetic glucocorticoid	A. Acromegaly
_____ Derived from arachidonic acid	B. Adenohypophysis
_____ Premature aging that occurs in childhood	C. Adenoma
_____ Caused by a deficient quantity of ADH	D. Cushing's syndrome
_____ Used to treat decreased activity of the thyroid	E. Diabetes insipidus
_____ Excessive thirst	F. Diabetes mellitus
_____ Caused by excessive growth hormone in adult	G. Levothyroxine sodium
_____ Posterior portion of the pituitary gland	H. Myxedema
_____ Tumor of a gland	I. Neurohypophysis
_____ A group of symptoms caused by prolonged exposure to high levels of cortisol	J. Polydipsia
	K. Polyphagia
	L. Prednisone
	M. Prostaglandins
	N. Progeria

2. Write the meaning of the following abbreviations.

_____ ACTH

_____ ADH

_____ DKA

_____ FSH

_____ IDDM

3. Spelling is important in scientific and medical applications because only one or two incorrect letters may change the meaning. All of the following words are from this chapter and are spelled incorrectly. Write the correct spelling in the space preceding the misspelled words.

_____ epinefrin

_____ hydrocloric

_____ natrietic

_____ prostraglandins

_____ lutinizing

4. Write the meaning of the underlined portion of each word on the line preceding the word.

_____ an<u>dro</u>gen

_____ endo<u>crine</u>

_____ prog<u>este</u>rone

_____ <u>pine</u>al

_____ oxy<u>toc</u>in

_____ <u>acro</u>megaly

_____ acro<u>megaly</u>

_____ ad<u>renal</u>

_____ <u>ad</u>renal

_____ <u>para</u>thyroid

5. Using your knowledge of word parts, match the following terms and definitions.

_____	Inflammation of the pancreas	A. Adrenalectomy
_____	Surgical removal of the pituitary gland	B. Adrenalitis
_____	Tumor of the pineal gland	C. Endocrinopathy
_____	Any disorder of the endocrine system	D. Hypophysectomy
_____	Surgical removal of an adrenal gland	E. Pancreatalgia
_____	Inflammation of the adrenal gland	F. Pancreatitis
_____	Pain in the pancreas	G. Pinealoma
_____	Enlargement of the thyroid gland	H. Thyromegaly

FUN AND GAMES

This is a variation of the word game of Hangman. Guess any letter for the first word and find the number that corresponds to that letter in the Letter Chart at the bottom of the page. Then find that same number above the line that divides each cell in the Position Chart on the right. If the letter you guessed appears in the word, its position is given by the number or numbers below the line that divides each cell in the Position Chart. If the letter does not appear in the word, 0 will be indicated under the line. If the letter you guessed does not appear in the word, start drawing a stick person on a gallows – first a head, then a body, followed by two arms and two legs. You are allotted six wrong guesses before you are hanged. Clue: All words are hormones.

Words

#1 _ _ _ _ _ _ _ _ _ _ _ _
   1 2 3 4 5 6 7 8 9 10 11 12

#2 _ _ _ _ _ _ _ _ _
   1 2 3 4 5 6 7 8 9

#3 _ _ _ _ _ _ _ _
   1 2 3 4 5 6 7 8

#4 _ _ _ _ _ _ _ _ _ _
   1 2 3 4 5 6 7 8 9 10

#5 _ _ _ _ _ _ _ _ _ _ _
   1 2 3 4 5 6 7 8 9 10 11

#6 _ _ _ _ _ _ _ _ _ _ _ _
   1 2 3 4 5 6 7 8 9 10 11 12

#7 _ _ _ _ _ _ _
   1 2 3 4 5 6 7

#8 _ _ _ _ _ _ _ _
   1 2 3 4 5 6 7 8

#9 _ _ _ _ _ _ _ _
   1 2 3 4 5 6 7 8

#10 _ _ _ _ _ _ _ _ _ _ _ _
   1 2 3 4 5 6 7 8 9 10 11 12

Letters Missed

| _ | _ | _ | _ | _ | _ |

| _ | _ | _ | _ | _ | _ |

| _ | _ | _ | _ | _ | _ |

| _ | _ | _ | _ | _ | _ |

| _ | _ | _ | _ | _ | _ |

| _ | _ | _ | _ | _ | _ |

| _ | _ | _ | _ | _ | _ |

| _ | _ | _ | _ | _ | _ |

| _ | _ | _ | _ | _ | _ |

| _ | _ | _ | _ | _ | _ |

Position Chart

1	2	3	4	5
6	9	9	7	1, 6
6	**7**	**8**	**9**	**10**
2	1, 5	1	8	2, 8, 12
11	**12**	**13**	**14**	**15**
4	1, 7	1, 4	3, 6	7, 10
16	**17**	**18**	**19**	**20**
0	1	7	4	7
21	**22**	**23**	**24**	**25**
8, 3	0	2	11	4, 9
26	**27**	**28**	**29**	**30**
0	8	2	2, 9	9
31	**32**	**33**	**34**	**35**
0	8	5	4	2
36	**37**	**38**	**39**	**40**
1, 6	4	0	5, 9	0
41	**42**	**43**	**44**	**45**
5	6	4	6	6
46	**47**	**48**	**49**	**50**
4	0	11	0	3
51	**52**	**53**	**54**	**55**
12	3	5	8, 10	10
56	**57**	**58**	**59**	**60**
7	0	1, 4, 7	3	3, 10
61	**62**	**63**	**64**	**65**
6	2, 7	3	8	3
66	**67**	**68**	**69**	**70**
8	0	0	7, 11	6
71	**72**	**73**	**74**	**75**
1	1	7	5	2, 4
76	**77**	**78**	**79**	**80**
5, 8, 12	5	5	6	3
81	**82**	**83**	**84**	**85**
11	5, 10	2	3	2

Letter Chart

	A	B	C	D	E	F	G	H	I	J	K	L	M	N	O	P	Q	R	S	T	U	V	W	X	Y	Z
#1	75	16	68	38	51	26	67	42	22	47	68	31	3	81	15	72	40	21	68	33	49	16	38	57	26	47
#2	41	38	79	22	31	40	49	67	66	16	31	11	47	2	59	17	26	85	16	20	38	67	26	49	16	31
#3	16	26	70	38	47	67	22	38	4	49	68	26	40	27	7	67	57	47	38	46	22	40	68	35	84	26
#4	83	57	13	68	16	57	16	31	39	47	67	65	22	54	73	26	38	31	47	1	16	26	31	47	57	22
#5	71	22	31	50	69	38	49	68	26	40	57	6	16	55	25	49	68	32	77	45	31	49	22	67	31	68
#6	40	49	67	16	10	31	47	67	22	38	49	68	26	24	82	47	57	30	14	58	26	38	16	57	22	38
#7	26	38	47	57	68	40	57	16	5	31	47	74	67	62	16	22	38	40	52	22	19	22	31	40	49	67
#8	78	16	34	31	47	22	36	38	49	68	26	23	40	64	56	26	31	57	16	49	63	26	38	47	68	16
#9	67	22	38	49	12	57	61	16	31	47	67	22	38	9	53	38	67	43	28	80	16	22	31	40	49	26
#10	68	26	40	57	76	49	37	68	26	40	57	16	38	48	60	8	16	29	44	18	38	47	57	26	67	38

11
Blood

KEY TERMS

Agglutinin
Agglutinogen
Coagulation
Diapedesis
Erythrocyte
Erythropoiesis
Erythropoietin
Hemocytoblast
Hemopoiesis
Leukocyte
Thrombocyte

BUILDING VOCABULARY

agglutin-
anti-
coagul-
-emia
erythr-
fibr-
glob-
hem-
kary-
leuk-
-lysis
mon-
-penia
-pheresis
-phil
plast-
-poiesis
poikil-
-rrhage
-stasis
thromb-

CLINICAL TERMS

Anemia
Coagulopathy
Ecchymosis
Embolus
Erythrocytosis
Hematocrit
Hemophilia
Leukocytosis
Leukopenia
Multiple myeloma
Petechia
Plasmapheresis
Polycythemia
Purpura
Reticulocyte
Thrombocytopenia
Thrombus

CLINICAL ABBREVIATIONS

AML
CBC
CML
DIC
ESR
Hb
HCT
MCH
PCV
PMN
PT
RBC
Rh
segs
WBC

OUTLINE/OBJECTIVES

Functions and Characteristics of Blood

- Describe the physical characteristics and functions of blood.
  — Blood is a liquid connective tissue; measures about 5 liters; accounts for 8% body weight; is slightly heavier than water; is 4 to 5 times more viscous than water; and has a pH of 7.35 to 7.45.
  — Blood transports gases, nutrients, and waste products; helps regulate body temperature, fluid and electrolyte balance, pH; helps prevent fluid loss and disease.

Composition of Blood

- Describe the composition of blood plasma.
  — Blood is 55% plasma and 45% formed elements.
  — Plasma is 90% water; the remaining 10% includes various solutes such as plasma proteins, gases, electrolytes, nutrients, and other molecules.
  — Plasma proteins include the albumins, globulins, and fibrinogen. Albumins account for 60% of the plasma proteins. They maintain the osmotic pressure of the blood. Globulins account for 36% of the plasma proteins. They function in lipid transport and in immune reactions. Fibrinogen accounts for 4% of the plasma proteins. It functions in the formation of blood clots.
  — Amino acids, urea, and uric acid are nonprotein molecules that contain nitrogen and may be present in blood plasma.
  — Simple nutrients that are the end products of digestion are transported in the plasma.
  — Oxygen and carbon dioxide are gases that are transported in the plasma.
  — Sodium, potassium, calcium, chloride, bicarbonate, and phosphate ions are common electrolytes in the blood plasma. Electrolytes contribute to the osmotic pressure of the blood, maintain membrane potentials, and regulate pH of body fluids.
- Identify the formed elements of the blood and state at least one function for each formed element.
  — Three categories of formed elements are erythrocytes, leukocytes, and thrombocytes.
  — Erythrocytes (red blood cells, RBC) are anucleate, biconcave disks, about 7.5 μm in diameter; there are 4.5–6 million/mm^3 blood; they contain hemoglobin. The primary function of erythrocytes is to transport oxygen.
  — Leukocytes (white blood cells, WBCs) have a nucleus and do not have hemoglobin; they average between 5000/mm^3 and 9000/mm^3; they move through capillary walls by diapedesis. WBCs provide a defense against disease and mediate inflammatory reactions.
  — Thrombocytes, or platelets, are fragments of megakaryocytes that function in blood clotting; they average 250,000–500,000/mm^3 of blood.
- Discuss the life cycle of erythrocytes.
  — Erythrocyte production is regulated by erythropoietin, which is activated by renal erythropoietin factor. Iron, vitamin B$_{12}$, and folic acid are essential for RBC production.
  — The life span of RBCs is about 120 days; then they are destroyed by the spleen and liver. The iron and protein portions are reused; the pigment portion is converted to bilirubin and is secreted in bile.
- Differentiate between five types of leukocytes on the basis of their structure.
  — Neutrophils are granulocytes with light-colored granules; they are the most numerous leukocyte and are phagocytic.
  — Eosinophils are granulocytes with red granules; they help counteract the effects of histamine.

— Basophils are granulocytes with blue granules; they secrete histamine and heparin. In the tissues they are called mast cells.
— Lymphocytes are agranulocytes that have a special role in immune processes; some attack bacteria directly, others produce antibodies.
— Monocytes are large phagocytic agranulocytes. In the tissues they are called macrophages.

Hemostasis

- Describe the mechanisms that reduce blood loss after trauma.
  — Hemostasis, the stoppage of bleeding, includes vascular constriction, platelet plug formation, and coagulation.
  — The initial reaction in hemostasis is vascular constriction, which reduces the flow of blood through a torn or severed vessel.
  — Collagen from damaged tissues attracts platelets, which form a platelet plug to fill the gap in a broken vessel to reduce blood loss.
  — Coagulation, or blood clot formation, starts with the formation of prothrombin activator, continues with the conversion of prothrombin to thrombin, and ends with the conversion of soluble fibrinogen to insoluble fibrin. Calcium and vitamin K are necessary for successful clot formation. After a clot forms, it condenses, or retracts, to pull the edges of the wound together. As healing takes place, the clot dissolves by fibrinolysis.

Blood Typing and Transfusions

- Characterize the different blood types and explain why some are incompatible for transfusions.
  — Blood type antigens on the surface of RBCs are called agglutinogens. Antibodies that react with agglutinogens are in the plasma and are called agglutinins.
  — The ABO blood types are based on the agglutinogens present on the surface of the RBCs. Type A blood has type A agglutinogens and anti-B agglutinins; type B blood has type B agglutinogens and anti-A agglutinins; type AB blood has both type A and type B agglutinogens but neither agglutinin; type O blood has neither agglutinogen but has both anti-A and anti-B agglutinins.
  — In transfusion reactions involving mismatched blood, the recipient's agglutinins react with the donor's agglutinogens. Type AB blood is called the universal recipient and type O is the universal donor.
  — People who have Rh+ blood have Rh agglutinogens; Rh− individuals do not have Rh agglutinogens. Normally, neither type has anti-Rh agglutinins. Exposure to Rh+ blood causes an Rh− individual to develop anti-Rh agglutinins and subsequent exposures may result in a transfusion reaction.
  — Hemolytic disease of the newborn is a threat when the mother is Rh− and the developing fetus is Rh+. If the mother has previously developed anti-Rh agglutinins, they may cross the placenta and enter the fetal blood, causing agglutination and hemolysis. If hemolytic disease of the newborn develops, the fetal blood is temporarily replaced with Rh− blood.

LEARNING EXERCISES

Functions and Characteristics of Blood

1. Write the terms that best fit the following phrases about the functions and characteristics of blood.

_____	pH range of the blood
_____	Normal volume of blood
_____	Types of substances transported by blood (3)
_____	
_____	
_____	Regulatory functions of blood (3)
_____	
_____	

Composition of Blood

1. The following statement is false. Rewrite the stateme\nt to make it true. Blood is 70% plasma and 30% formed elements.

2. Complete the following table about plasma proteins.

Plasma Protein	Percent of Total	Function
	60%	
Globulin		
		Blood clotting

3. Give two examples for each of the following plasma components.

Nonprotein molecules that contain nitrogen _____

_____

Nutrients _____

_____

Gases _____

_____

Electrolytes _____

_____

4. Write the scientific term for each of the three types of formed elements in the blood.

   Red blood cells _____

   White blood cells _____

   Platelets _____

5. Identify each of the formed elements illustrated in the following diagram by matching the letters with the names. Color the granulocytes yellow and color the agranulocytes green.

   _____ Basophil

   _____ Eosinophil

   _____ Erythrocyte

   _____ Lymphocyte

   _____ Monocyte

   _____ Neutrophil

6. Write the terms that best fit the following phrases about the formed elements of blood.

   _____ Anucleate biconcave disks

   _____ Immature RBCs circulating in the blood

   _____ Normal range of RBCs/mm^3 in blood

   _____ Large protein pigment in RBCs

   _____ Process by which WBCs enter tissue spaces

   _____ Normal range of WBCs/mm^3 in blood

   _____ Most numerous leukocyte

   _____ Leukocyte with red-staining granules

   _____ Contains histamine and heparin

   _____ Largest leukocyte

   _____ Function in antibody production

_____	Multilobed nucleus
_____	Called macrophages in the tissues
_____	Phagocytic granulocyte
_____	Phagocytic agranulocyte
_____	Called mast cells in the tissues
_____	Help counteract effects of histamine
_____	Function of thrombocytes
_____	Normal range of platelets/mm^3 in the blood
_____	Cell that breaks apart to form platelets

7. Write the terms that best fit the following phrases about erythrocyte production.

_____	Stem cell in the bone marrow
_____	Hormone that stimulates RBC production
_____	Mineral necessary for healthy RBCs
_____	Vitamins necessary for RBC production (2)
_____	
_____	Necessary for absorption of vitamin B_{12}
_____	Average life span of RBCs
_____	Organs where old RBCs are phagocytized (2)
_____	
_____	Waste product of RBC destruction

Hemostasis

1. Write the terms that best fit the following phrases about hemostasis.

_____	Initial reaction in hemostasis
_____	Process of collagen attracting platelets
_____	Vitamin necessary for clot formation
_____	Mineral necessary for clot formation
_____	Dissolution of a clot

2. The following diagram shows three reactions in blood clotting. Identify substances A, B, C, and D.

Damaged Tissues ⟶ Formation of Substance A

Substance B ⟶ Substance C

Substance D ⟶ Fibrin

Substance A _____   Substance C _____

Substance B _____   Substance D _____

Blood Typing and Transfusions

1. Complete the following table about the different ABO blood types. For the permissible donor column, assume that a person with the given blood type needs a transfusion and the preferred type is not available. What are the other possible donor types? For the permissible recipient column, what blood types may receive the indicated type if the preferred type is not available?

Blood Type	Agglutinogen	Agglutinin	Permissible Donors	Permissible Recipients
A				
	B			
		None		
	None			

2. Write the terms that best fit the following phrases about Rh+ and Rh− blood.

_____ Agglutinogen in Rh+ blood

_____ Agglutinogen in Rh− blood

_____ Agglutinin in unsensitized Rh+ blood

_____ Agglutinin in unsensitized Rh− blood

3. Answer the following questions about Rh+ and Rh− blood.

What happens if an unsensitized Rh− individual receives Rh+ blood?

What happens if a sensitized Rh− individual receives Rh+ blood?

An Rh+ individual does not develop anti-Rh antibodies after receiving Rh− blood. Why?

What maternal and fetal blood types may lead to hemolytic disease of the newborn?

Maternal type:

Fetal type:

REVIEW QUESTIONS

1. What is the total volume of blood in the human body? What is its normal pH?

2. Name five substances that are transported in the blood.

3. In addition to transport, what are five other functions of the blood?

4. What percentage of the blood is plasma? What percentage is formed elements?

5. What is the major component of plasma?

6. What are the three major plasma proteins and what is the function of each?

7. Identify three types of formed elements, their precursor cells, and the process by which they are formed.

8. Describe the physical characteristics of erythrocytes and state the normal number.

9. What is the primary function of erythrocytes and what molecule within the erythrocyte carries out this function?

10. How is the production of erythrocytes regulated and what three factors are necessary for normal production?

11. What is the normal life span of an erythrocyte and what happens to its components when it is destroyed?

12. How do the physical characteristics of leukocytes differ from those of erythrocytes?

13. Identify three granulocytes and two agranulocytes and state the function of each one. Which one is most numerous? Which one is least numerous?

14. What are thrombocytes and what is their function? How many are normally present in the blood?

15. Define hemostasis and describe each of the three processes that contribute to hemostasis.

16. Write three word equations that summarize the steps in coagulation of blood.

17. Name an ion and a vitamin that are necessary for coagulation.

18. As healing progresses, what happens to a blood clot?

19. What agglutinogens and agglutinins are present in each of the five ABO blood types?

20. How do the agglutinogens and agglutinins react in a mismatched transfusion?

21. What ABO blood type is called the universal donor? What type is the universal recipient? Why?

22. What distinguishes Rh+ individuals from Rh− individuals?

23. What happens when an Rh− individual is first exposed to Rh+ blood? What happens when exposed a second time?

24. What is hemolytic disease of the newborn? How does it develop?

25. How is hemolytic disease of the newborn treated? How can it be prevented?

CHAPTER QUIZ

1. Which one of the following is *not* true about blood? (a) the normal volume of blood is about 5 liters; (b) the normal pH is slightly acidic; (c) blood helps regulate body temperature; (d) blood is classified as a connective tissue; (e) blood is more viscous than water

2. Which of the following statements about plasma is *not* true? (a) plasma is about 90% water; (b) fibrinogen is a plasma protein that functions in clotting; (c) the most abundant plasma proteins are the globulins; (d) bicarbonate ions are found as solutes in the plasma; (e) some oxygen and carbon dioxide are transported as solutes in the plasma

3. Write the terms that best fit each of the following.

   _____ Production of formed elements

   _____ The stem cell from which blood cells develop

   _____ Hemoglobin that is combined with oxygen

   _____ Most numerous type of leukocyte

   _____ Hormone that stimulates RBC production

   _____ Process of WBCs moving through capillary walls

   _____ Leukocyte that produces antibodies

4. Indicate whether each of the following pertains to erythrocytes (E), leukocytes (L), or thrombocytes (T).

   _____ Fragments of large cells

   _____ Contain hemoglobin

   _____ May have granules in the cytoplasm

   _____ Some are phagocytic

   _____ Biconcave disks

   _____ Platelets

   _____ Transport oxygen

   _____ Primary function is blood clotting

   _____ Function in prevention of disease

   _____ Normal number is about 5 million/mm^3

5. Number the following events of hemostasis in the sequence in which they occur. The first event is 1 and the final event is 5.

   _____ Prothrombin is converted to thrombin

   _____ Smooth muscle in vessel walls contracts

   _____ Formation of prothrombin activator

   _____ Fibrinogen is converted to fibrin

   _____ Collagen attracts platelets to form platelet plug

6. Indicate whether each of the following pertains to blood type A, B, AB, or O. Some may have more than one answer.

_____   Has anti-A agglutinins

_____   Can be given to type B individuals

_____   Has no agglutinogens

_____   Universal recipient

_____   Has no agglutinins

_____   Can be given to type O individuals

_____   Can donate to type A individuals

_____   Has type B agglutinogens

_____   Universal donor

_____   Reacts with type AB donor blood

7. Which of the following statements about Rh blood types is *not* true? (a) about 85% of the population is Rh+; (b) normally, Rh− individuals do not have anti-Rh agglutinins; (c) normally, Rh+ individuals do not have anti-Rh agglutinins; (d) normally, Rh− individuals have Rh agglutinogens; (e) normally, Rh+ individuals have Rh agglutinogens

8. Indicate whether each of the following statements is true or false.

_____   When Rh− blood is given to an Rh+ individual, the Rh+ individual develops anti-Rh agglutinins.

_____   When Rh+ blood is given to an Rh− individual, the Rh− individual develops anti-Rh agglutinogens.

_____   Hemolytic disease of the newborn may develop when the mother is Rh− and the fetus is Rh+.

_____   Hemolytic disease of the newborn causes agglutination and hemolysis of the fetal blood.

_____   If hemolytic disease of the newborn develops, the fetus should receive a transfusion of Rh+ blood.

USING CLINICAL KNOWLEDGE

1. Match the definitions on the left with the correct term from the column on the right by placing the corresponding letter in the space before the definition. Not all terms will be used.

_____ On the surface of RBCs		A. Agglutinin
_____ Stem cell in the bone marrow		B. Agglutinogen
_____ Blood clot		C. Antihemophilic factors
_____ Multiple pinpoint hemorrhages		D. Coumadin
_____ An increase in the number of RBCs		E. Hematocrit
_____ Malignant tumor of bone marrow		F. Hemocytoblast
_____ Percentage of RBCs in whole blood		G. Heparin
_____ Immature RBC		H. Multiple myeloma
_____ Replace clotting factors absent from blood		I. Polycythemia
_____ Oral anticoagulant that prevents synthesis of clotting factors		J. Purpura
		K. Reticulocyte
		L. Thrombus

2. Write the meaning of the following abbreviations.

_____ CBC

_____ PCV

_____ Hb

_____ HCT

_____ Rh

3. Spelling is important in scientific and medical applications because only one or two incorrect letters may change the meaning. All of the following words are from this chapter and are spelled incorrectly. Write the correct spelling in the space preceding the misspelled words.

_____ dipedesis

_____ lukosites

_____ hemopoesis

_____ agllutination

_____ hemolitic

4. Write the meaning of the underlined portion of each word on the line preceding the word.

_____ erythro̲cyte

_____ megakary̲ocyte

_____ thrombo̲cyte

_____ mega̲karyocyte

_____ erythro<u>cyte</u>

_____ thrombocyto<u>penia</u>

_____ erythro<u>poietin</u>

_____ baso<u>phil</u>

_____ hemo<u>stasis</u>

_____ <u>agglutin</u>ogen

FUN AND GAMES

Each of the following terms is taken from this chapter and pertains to the blood in some way. The words also contain people's names with the letters in the correct sequence but there may be additional letters between the letters of the name. Fill in the spaces around the thirty names to complete the terms.

P _ A _ M _

F O R _ _ D _ _ _ _ _ _ _

_ R _ _ _ _ O _ Y _ _

_ L O _ U _ _ _

E _ _ _ _ R _ _ _ I _ _ _ N

_ _ _ _ _ _ T I N A _ _ _ _

L _ U _ _ C Y _ _

_ _ S T A _ _ N _

_ _ B _ _ _ _ _ E N

_ _ _ _ _ _ _ _ _ _ _ M I A

_ G _ L _ _ _ _ _ _ E N

_ _ R O _ B _ _

L _ _ _ _ O _ _ T _

D _ A _ _ D E _ _ _

M A _ R _ _ _ _ G E

_ _ _ _ _ _ _ P H I L

A _ _ _ _ _ _ _ N _ N

_ R O _ _ _ _ _ B I N

N E _ _ _ _ _ _ I L

M A _ _ C _ _ _ _

P _ _ A T _ _ _ _

_ _ S O P H I _

B _ _ _ R U _ I N

M _ _ A _ R _ _ C Y _ _

G R A _ _ _ _ C _ _ E

_ _ M A _ _ _ R I _

T _ _ O M _ _ _ _ _ _

A L _ _ _ _ _ _

A _ R _ _ _ _ _ _ _ _ T _

_ A _ _ _ _ L _ B _ _ I N

KEY TERMS

Atrioventricular valve
Cardiac cycle
Cardiac output
Conduction myofibers
Diastole
Semilunar valve
Stroke volume
Systole

BUILDING VOCABULARY

aort-
atri-
brady-
cardi-
coron-
cusp-
diastol-
ech-
lun-
meg-
sept-
son-
sphygm-
sten-
steth-
systol-
tachy-
valvu-

CLINICAL TERMS

Angina pectoris
Artificial pacemaker
Auscultation

Cardiac arrest
Cardiac catheterization
Cardiomegaly
Cardiomyopathy
Congestive heart failure
Coronary artery bypass grafting
Cor pulmonale
Defibrillation
Echocardiography
Fibrillation
Heart block
Mitral valve prolapse
Myocardial infarction
Valvular heart disease

CLINICAL ABBREVIATIONS

AI
ASD
ASHD
AV
CABG
CAD
CHF
CPR
LA
LCA
LV
MI
MVP
NTG
PVC
RA
RCA
RV
SA
VSD

OUTLINE/OBJECTIVES

Overview of the Heart

- Describe the size and location of the heart.
  - The heart, about the size of a closed fist, is located in the middle mediastinum between the second and sixth ribs. The apex points downward and to the left so that 2/3 of the mass is on the left side.
  - The heart is enclosed in a double-layered pericardial sac. The outer layer is fibrous connective tissue. The inner layer is parietal serous membrane. The visceral layer of the serous membrane forms the surface of the heart and is called the epicardium. The space between the parietal and visceral layers of the serous membrane is the pericardial cavity.

Structure of the Heart

- Identify the layers of the heart wall and state the type of tissue in each layer.
  - The outermost layer of the heart wall is the visceral layer of the serous pericardium and is called the epicardium.
  - The middle layer of the heart wall is the cardiac muscle tissue. It is the thickest layer and is called the myocardium.
  - The innermost layer is simple squamous epithelium and is called the endocardium.
- Label a diagram of the heart, identifying the chambers, valves, and associated vessels.
  - The right atrium is a thin-walled chamber that receives deoxygenated blood from the superior vena cava, inferior vena cava, and coronary sinus.
  - The right ventricle receives blood from the right atrium and pumps it out to the lungs to receive oxygen. It has a thick myocardium.
  - The left atrium is a thin-walled chamber that receives oxygenated blood from the lungs through the pulmonary veins.
  - The left ventricle has the thickest myocardium. It receives the oxygenated blood from the left atrium and pumps it out to systemic circulation.
  - There are two types of valves associated with the heart: atrioventricular (AV) valves and semilunar valves. AV valves are located between the atria and ventricles and prevent blood from flowing back into the atria when the ventricles contract. Semilunar valves are located at the exists from the ventricles and prevent blood from flowing back into the ventricles when the ventricles relax.
  - The AV valve on the right side is the tricuspid valve. On the left, it is the bicuspid, or mitral, valve. The pulmonary semilunar valve is located at the exit of the right ventricle. The aortic semilunar valve is at the exit of the left ventricle.
- Trace the pathway of blood flow through the heart, including chambers, valves, and pulmonary circulation.
  - Deoxygenated blood enters the right atrium through the superior vena cava, inferior vena cava, and coronary sinus. From the right atrium, the blood goes through the tricuspid valve into the right ventricle, then is pumped through the pulmonary semilunar valve into the pulmonary trunk, then pulmonary arteries, to the capillaries of the lungs. In the lung capillaries, the blood gives off CO_2, picks up O_2, then enters the pulmonary veins, and flows into the left atrium.
  - Oxygenated blood in the left atrium goes through the bicuspid valve into the left ventricle, then is pumped through the aortic semilunar valve into the ascending aorta to enter systemic circulation.
- Identify the major vessels that supply blood to the myocardium and return the deoxygenated blood to the right atrium.

— The right and left coronary arteries, branches of the ascending aorta, supply blood to the myocardium in the wall of the heart.

— Blood from the capillaries in the myocardium enters the cardiac veins, which drain into the coronary sinus. From there it enters the right atrium.

Physiology of the Heart

- Describe the components and function of the conduction system of the heart.
  - The conduction system of the heart consists of specialized cardiac muscle cells that act in a manner similar to neural tissue. The conduction system coordinates the contraction and relaxation of the heart chambers.
  - The sinoatrial (SA) node has the fastest rate of depolarization; therefore, it is the pacemaker in the conduction system. Other components in the conduction system are the AV node, AV bundle, bundle branches, and conduction myofibers.
  - An electrocardiogram is a recording of the electrical activity of the heart. The P wave is produced by depolarization of the atrial myocardium. The QRS wave is produced by depolarization of the ventricular myocardium and repolarization of the atria. The T wave is due to repolarization of the ventricles.
- Summarize the events of a complete cardiac cycle and correlate the heart sounds heard with a stethoscope with these events.
  - Systole is the contraction phase of the cardiac cycle and diastole is the relaxation phase. At a normal heart rate, one complete cardiac cycle lasts for 0.8 sec. Atrial systole lasts for 0.1 sec. followed by ventricular systole for 0.3 sec. All chambers are in diastole at the same time for 0.4 sec. Most ventricular filling occurs while all chambers are relaxed.
  - Heart sounds are due to vibrations in the blood caused by the valves closing. The first heart sound is caused by closure of the AV valves. The second heart sound is caused by closure of the semilunar valves.
- Explain what is meant by stroke volume and cardiac output and describe the factors that affect these values.
  - Cardiac output equals stroke volume times heart rate. Anything that affects either component affects the output.
  - Stroke volume is the amount of blood ejected from the ventricles during one cardiac cycle. It is influenced by end-diastolic volume and contraction strength. End-diastolic volume depends on venous return and contraction strength depends on end-diastolic volume and stimulation by the autonomic nervous system.
  - Heart rate directly influences cardiac output. The cardiac center in the medulla oblongata has both sympathetic and parasympathetic components that adjust the heart rate to meet the changing needs of the body. Peripheral baroreceptors and chemoreceptors send impulses to the cardiac center where appropriate responses adjust heart rate. Emotions and body temperature also affect heart rate. These effects are usually coordinated through the cardiac center.

LEARNING EXERCISES

Overview of the Heart

1. All of the following statements are false. Rewrite each statement to make it true.

   The base of the heart is directed inferiorly and to the left.

About 1/3 of the heart mass is on the left side.

The heart is located in the anterior mediastinum, between the second and fifth ribs.

2. Arrange the following coverings around the heart in the correct sequence by numbering them in the order in which they occur. Start with 1 for the outermost layer and proceed to 4 for the innermost layer.

_____ Epicardium

_____ Fibrous pericardium

_____ Pericardial cavity

_____ Parietal pericardium

Structure of the Heart

1. Write the terms that best fit the following phrases about the structure of the heart.

_____ Middle layer of the heart wall

_____ Chamber that receives blood from the superior vena cava

_____ Valve between the right atrium and ventricle

_____ Inner lining of the heart wall

_____ Receives oxygenated blood from the lungs

_____ Thin region of the interatrial septum

_____ Receives blood from the right atrium

_____ Ridges of myocardium in the ventricles

_____ Atrioventricular valve on left side of the heart

_____ Valve at base of the aorta

_____ Arteries that supply blood to the myocardium

_____ Chamber that receives blood from the inferior vena cava

2. Identify the listed structures of the heart by matching them with the correct letters from the diagram. Use blue to color the chambers and vessels that contain oxygen-poor blood. Use red to color the chambers and vessels that contain oxygen-rich blood.

_____ Right atrium

_____ Right ventricle

_____ Left atrium

_____ Left ventricle

_____ Interventricular septum

_____ Superior vena cava

_____ Inferior vena cava

_____ Pulmonary trunk

_____ Ascending aorta

_____ Right brachiocephalic vein

_____ Brachiocephalic artery

_____ Aortic semilunar valve

_____ Pulmonary semilunar valve

_____ Tricuspid valve

_____ Bicuspid valve

_____ Left common carotid artery

_____ Left subclavian artery

_____ Left pulmonary artery

3. Trace the pathway of blood through the heart by numbering the following structures in the correct sequence. Start with number 1 for the venae cavae.

_____ Aortic semilunar valve

_____ Ascending aorta

_____ Bicuspid valve

_____ Capillaries of lungs

_____ Left atrium

_____ Left ventricle

_____ Pulmonary semilunar valve

_____ Pulmonary trunk

_____ Pulmonary veins

_____ Pulmonary arteries

_____ Right atrium

_____ Right ventricle

_____ Tricuspid valve

_____ Venae cavae

Physiology of the Heart

1. Write the terms that best fit the following phrases about the conduction system of the heart and the cardiac cycle.

    _____ Pacemaker of the heart

    _____ Length of cardiac cycle at 72 beats/minute

    _____ Indicates depolarization of the atria on ECG

    _____ Transmits impulses to the atria and AV node

    _____ A recording of the electrical activity of the heart

    _____ Indicates depolarization of ventricles on ECG

    _____ Contraction phase of the ventricles

    _____ Carry impulses to the myocardium

    _____ Indicates repolarization of the ventricles on ECG

    _____ Relaxation phase of the ventricles

    _____ Transmit impulses away from the AV node

    _____ Length of atrial systole in one cardiac cycle

    _____ Normally has fastest rate of depolarization

    _____ Length of ventricular systole in one cycle

2. In the space before each phrase about events in the cardiac cycle, write S if the phrase refers to ventricular systole and write D if it refers to ventricular diastole.

    _____ Atria are in systole   _____ Semilunar (SL) valves close

    _____ Atrioventricular (AV)   _____ Blood is ejected from
            valves open   the heart

    _____ Atrioventricular (AV)   _____ Pressure in ventricles
            valves close   decreases

    _____ Semilunar (SL) valves open   _____ Blood enters the ventricles

3. Heart sounds are associated with heart valves closing. Which valves are associated with the following sounds?

    (a) First heart sound (lubb)

    (b) Second heart sound (dupp)

4. In the space before each statement about factors that influence cardiac output, write T if the statement is true and write F if the statement is false. If the statement is false, change the underlined word(s) to make the statement true.

_____   Cardiac output equals heart rate <u>plus</u> stroke volume.

_____   Stroke volume is the amount of blood ejected from the heart during each <u>cardiac cycle</u>.

_____   Increased venous return <u>decreases</u> contraction strength.

_____   Sympathetic stimulation <u>decreases</u> contraction strength.

_____   Increased contraction strength <u>increases</u> cardiac output.

_____   Parasympathetic nerves <u>decrease</u> heart rate.

_____   Increased end-diastolic volume <u>decreases</u> stroke volume.

_____   Sympathetic stimulation <u>increases</u> heart rate.

_____   Increased end-diastolic volume <u>increases</u> cardiac output.

_____   Most changes in heart rate are mediated through the cardiac center in the <u>pons</u>.

_____   Epinephrine <u>decreases</u> heart rate.

_____   Increased carbon dioxide concentration in the tissues <u>increases</u> heart rate.

REVIEW QUESTIONS

1. Specifically where within the middle mediastinum is the heart located? Where is the apex? Where is the base?

2. What are the two main components, or layers, of the pericardial sac?

3. Where is the pericardial cavity?

4. What are the three layers of the heart wall?

5. What is the difference in structure between the atria and ventricles?

6. How does the structural difference in the heart chambers reflect their functional difference?

7. How do atrioventricular valves and semilunar valves differ in structure?

8. How does the structural difference between atrioventricular and semilunar valves reflect their functional difference?

9. Identify the chambers and valves of the heart on a diagram.

10. List, in sequence, the structures through which blood passes as it goes from the right atrium to the ascending aorta.

11. How does the myocardium receive the oxygen that is required for contraction?

12. What are the components of the conduction system of the heart? Why is a conduction system necessary?

13. How do the waves, or deflections, of an electrocardiogram relate to events in the conduction system?

14. What is meant by the terms systole and diastole?

15. What happens during each part of the cardiac cycle and how long does each part last?

16. How do heart sounds relate to events of the cardiac cycle?

17. How is cardiac output calculated?

18. By what mechanisms does end-diastolic volume affect stroke volume and cardiac output?

19. What center in the brain regulates the rate of the sinoatrial node? Through what pathway does this regulation occur?

CHAPTER QUIZ

1. Which one of the following is *not* true about the location of the heart? (a) it is located in the middle mediastinum; (b) 2/3 of the mass of the heart is on the left side; (c) the heart extends between the second and sixth ribs; (d) the base of the heart is the lowest portion; (e) the heart is about the size of a closed fist

2. True or False: The fibrous pericardium is the outermost layer of the heart wall.

3. Use the words epicardium, endocardium, and myocardium to write a description of the structure of the heart wall.

4. Indicate whether each of the following pertains to the right atrium (RA), right ventricle (RV), left atrium (LA), or left ventricle (LV). More than one response may apply.

    _____ Receives blood from the pulmonary veins

    _____ Pumps blood to the lungs

    _____ Contains unoxygenated blood

    _____ Contains papillary muscles

    _____ Receives blood from the inferior vena cava

    _____ Pumps blood through the aortic semilunar valve

    _____ Pumps blood into systemic circulation

    _____ Receives blood through the tricuspid valve

    _____ Coronary sinus opens into this chamber

    _____ Bicuspid valve is at the exit of this chamber

5. Name the two major branches of the left coronary artery.

6. Indicate whether each of the following statements is true (T) or false (F).

    _____ Atrial systole lasts longer than ventricular systole.

    _____ All chambers are in simultaneous diastole for half the cardiac cycle.

    _____ An increase in right ventricular pressure closes the tricuspid valve and opens the semilunar valve.

    _____ Most of the blood enters the ventricles during atrial systole.

    _____ The P wave on an electrocardiogram corresponds to atrial depolarization.

    _____ The first heart sound is heard when the semilunar valves open.

_____ The T wave on an electrocardiogram corresponds to atrial repolarization.

_____ Impulses travel throughout ventricular myocardium by conduction myofibers.

_____ Ventricular diastole lasts longer than atrial diastole.

_____ Blood is oxygenated before it enters the right ventricle.

7. If stroke volume is 65 ml and heart rate is 75 beats/minute, what is the cardiac output per minute?

8. Which of the following statements is *not* true about cardiac output? (a) increased venous return increases contraction strength; (b) increased parasympathetic stimulation increases cardiac output; (c) increased end-diastolic volume increases contraction strength; (d) increased end-diastolic volume increases cardiac output; (e) increased sympathetic stimulation increases heart rate

USING CLINICAL KNOWLEDGE

1. Match the definitions on the left with the correct term from the column on the right by placing the corresponding letter in the space before the definition. Not all terms will be used.

_____ Contraction phase of the cardiac cycle	A. Angina pectoris
_____ Enlargement of the heart	B. Atrioventricular
_____ Rapid, random, irregular, ineffectual heart contractions	C. Auscultation
_____ Any primary disease of heart muscle	D. Cardiac infarction
_____ Drug that increases strength and regularity of heart contractions	E. Cardiac output
_____ Volume of blood ejected from one ventricle during contraction	F. Cardiomegaly
_____ Using a stethoscope to listen to heart sounds	G. Cardiomyopathy
_____ Acute chest pain caused by decreased blood supply to heart muscle	H. Diastole
_____ A vasodilator used to relieve the pain of angina pectoris	I. Digitalis (Digoxin)
_____ Valves between the heart ventricles and output vessels	J. Fibrillation
	K. Nitroglycerine
	L. Semilunar
	M. Stroke volume
	N. Systole

2. Write the meaning of the following abbreviations.

_____ CABG

_____ PVC

_____ CPR

_____ VSD

_____ CHF

3. Spelling is important in scientific and medical applications because only one or two incorrect letters may change the meaning. All of the following words are from this chapter and are spelled incorrectly. Write the correct spelling in the space preceding the misspelled words.

_____ arhythmia

_____ infarcshun

_____ distole

_____ conjestive

_____ fosa ovalis

4. Write the meaning of the underlined portion of each word on the line preceding the word.

_____   epi<u>cardi</u>um

_____   <u>my</u>ocardium

_____   <u>sten</u>osis

_____   <u>tachy</u>cardia

_____   electrocardi<u>ogram</u>

_____   semi<u>lun</u>ar

_____   <u>sphygmo</u>manometer

_____   <u>coron</u>ary

_____   <u>echo</u>cardiogram

_____   <u>steth</u>oscope

FUN AND GAMES

Thirty-three terms relating to the heart are described below. Determine the term that fits each description, then place it in the correct position on the grid. The descriptions are arranged according to the number of letters in the correct response.

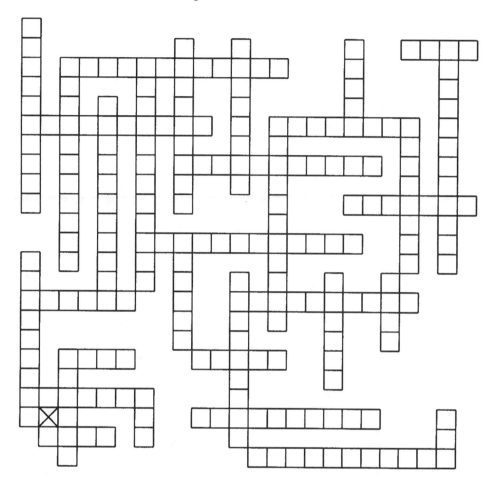

3 Letters
Heart activity record
Records ventricular contraction

4 Letters
Pointed end of the heart
End directed to the right
First heart sound
Second heart sound

5 Letters
Vessel exiting left ventricle
Returns blood to the heart

6 Letters
Thin-walled chamber
Heart pacemaker
Left AV valve
Takes blood away from heart

7 Letters
Contraction phase of cycle
Atrial appendage

8 Letters
Narrowing of an opening
Relaxation phase of cycle
Left AV valve

9 Letters
Pumping chamber of heart
Right AV valve
Valve at exit from heart

10 Letters
Outer layer of heart wall
Cardiac muscle layer
Inflammation of a valve
L coronary artery branch

11 Letters
Slow heart rate
Surrounds the heart
Innermost layer of wall
Thin area of septum
Rapid heart rate

12 Letters
Listening to the heart
Enlarged heart
Ejected during systole
Inflammation of lining

13

Blood Vessels

KEY TERMS

Diastolic pressure
Korotkoff sounds
Peripheral resistance
Pulse
Systolic pressure
Vasoconstriction
Vasodilation

BUILDING VOCABULARY

aneur-
angi-
arter-
ather-
brachi-
carot-
cephal-
edem-
embol-
isch-
phleb-
scler-
sten-
-tripsy
vas-
ven-

CLINICAL TERMS

Angiography
Angioplasty

Antiarrhythmic
Arterectomy
Arteriosclerosis
Antihypertensive
Atherectomy
Atheroma
Atherosclerosis
Hemangioma
Hemorrhoids
Hypoperfusion
Ischemia
Phlebitis
Phlebotomy
Raynaud's phenomenon
Varicose veins
Vasculitis

CLINICAL ABBREVIATIONS

ABP
ACE
CV
CVP
CSR
DSA
H&H
HBP
HPN
IVCP
KVO
PTA
PTCA
TEE

OUTLINE/OBJECTIVES

Classification and Structure of Blood Vessels

- Describe the structure and function of arteries, capillaries, and veins.
  — Arteries carry blood away from the heart. The wall of an artery consists of the tunica intima (simple squamous epithelium), tunica media (smooth muscle), and tunica externa (connective tissue).
  — Capillaries form the connection between arteries and veins. Their walls are simple squamous epithelium. Capillaries function in the exchange of materials between the blood and the tissue cells. The number of capillaries in a tissue depends on the metabolic activity of the tissue. Metabolically active tissues have an abundance of capillaries; less active tissues have fewer capillaries. Small arterioles and precapillary sphincters regulate blood flow into the capillaries.
  — Veins carry blood toward the heart. The walls of veins have the same three layers as the arteries, but the layers are thinner. Veins have valves to prevent the backflow of blood.

Physiology of Circulation

- Discuss how oxygen, carbon dioxide, glucose, and water move across capillary walls.
  — Oxygen, carbon dioxide, and glucose move across the capillary wall by simple diffusion.
  — Water moves across the capillary wall by filtration and osmosis.
- Discuss the factors that affect blood flow through arteries, capillaries, and veins.
  — Blood flows from a higher pressure area to a lower pressure area; it flows in the same direction as the pressure gradient.
  — Pressure is lowest as the venae cavae enter the right atrium. Pressure in the right atrium is called the central venous pressure.
  — Velocity of blood flow varies inversely with the total cross-sectional area of the blood vessels. As the area increases, the velocity decreases. Since capillaries are so numerous, they have the greatest cross-sectional area and the slowest blood flow.
  — Resistance is a force that opposes blood flow. As resistance increases, blood flow decreases. The autonomic nervous system regulates blood flow by changing the resistance of the vessels through vasoconstriction and vasodilation.
  — Very little pressure from ventricular contraction remains by the time the blood reaches the veins. Venous blood flow depends on skeletal muscle action, respiratory movements, and contraction of smooth muscle in venous walls.
- Describe the mechanisms and pressures that move gases and fluids across capillary walls.
  — Capillaries have a vital role in the exchange of gases, nutrients, and metabolic waste products between the blood and tissue cells. Solutes such as oxygen, carbon dioxide, and glucose move across the capillary wall by diffusion.
  — A combination of hydrostatic pressure and osmotic pressure determines fluid movement across the capillary wall. Fluid moves out of the capillary at the arteriole end and returns at the venous end.
- Discuss four primary factors that affect blood pressure and how blood pressure is regulated.
  — Pulse refers to the rhythmic expansion of an artery that is caused by ejection of blood from the ventricle. It can be felt where an artery is close to the surface and rests on something firm. These locations are called pulse points.
  — Systolic pressure is the pressure in the arteries during ventricular contraction (systole). Normal systolic pressure is about 120 mm Hg. Diastolic pressure is the pressure in the arteries during ventricular relaxation (diastole). Normal diastolic pressure is about 80 mm Hg. Pulse pressure is the difference between systolic pressure and diastolic pressure. This is usually

about 40 mm Hg. A sphygmomanometer is used to measure blood pressure. The brachial artery is a common site for measuring blood pressure. Cardiac output, blood volume, peripheral resistance, and viscosity of the blood affect blood pressure.

— Baroreceptors in the aortic arch and carotid sinus detect stretching in the vessel walls when blood pressure increases. Signals are relayed back to the heart and blood vessels that reduce the pressure. Baroreceptors are important in short-term blood pressure regulation.

— Chemoreceptors detect carbon dioxide, hydrogen ion, and oxygen concentrations. This is significant only in emergency situations.

— Antidiuretic hormone plays a role in regulating blood volume, which has an effect on blood pressure.

— In response to decreases in blood pressure, the kidneys secrete renin, which stimulates the production of angiotensin. Angiotensin causes vasoconstriction and promotes the release of aldosterone. Both actions result in increased blood pressure.

Circulatory Pathways

- Trace blood through the pulmonary circuit from the right atrium to the left atrium.
  — Pulmonary circulation transports oxygen-poor blood from the right ventricle to the lungs where the blood picks up a new blood supply then it returns the oxygen-rich blood to the left atrium. Figure 13-10 in the textbook shows the pathway of pulmonary circulation.
- Identify the major systemic arteries and veins.
  — Systemic arteries carry oxygenated blood from the left ventricle to the capillaries in the tissues of the body. Figures 13-11, 13-12, and 13-13 in the textbook illustrate the major systemic arteries.
  — Systemic veins carry oxygen-poor, carbon dioxide-laden blood from the tissues to the right atrium of the heart. Figures 13-15, 13-16, and 13-17 in the textbook illustrate the major systemic veins.
- Describe the blood supply to the brain.
  — The principal blood supply to the brain is through the internal carotid arteries and the vertebral arteries. Branches of these vessels form the circle of Willis at the base of the brain.
- Describe five features of fetal circulation that make it different from adult circulation.
  — There are some differences in the circulatory pathways of the fetus because the lungs, gastrointestinal tract, and kidneys are not functioning.
  — The two umbilical arteries carry fetal blood to the placenta; the umbilical vein carries blood from the placenta to the fetus; the placenta functions in the exchange of gases and nutrients between the maternal and fetal blood; the ductus venosus allows blood to bypass the immature fetal liver; the foramen ovale and ductus arteriosus permit blood to bypass the fetal lungs.

LEARNING EXERCISES

Classification and Structure of Blood Vessels

1. In the space before each phrase about blood vessels, write A if the phrase refers to an artery, C if it refers to a capillary, and V if it refers to a vein.

_____ Carries blood away from the heart

_____ Functions in the exchange of substances between blood and tissue cells

_____ Wall consists of simple squamous epithelium

_____   Carries blood toward the heart

_____   Has valves

_____   Has three relatively thick layers in the wall

_____   Has three relatively thin layers in the wall

_____   May have vasa vasorum

2. Name the tunic or layer in the wall of a blood vessel that contains predominantly

    (a) connective tissue

    (b) simple squamous epithelium

    (c) smooth muscle

Physiology of Circulation

1. Identify the passive transport process by which each of the following substances moves through the capillary wall.

    _____   Carbon dioxide

    _____   Oxygen

    _____   Water (2)

    _____

2. Write an A before the phrases that pertain to the arterial end of a capillary and write a V before the phrases that pertain to the venule end of a capillary.

    _____   Osmotic pressure is greater than hydrostatic pressure

    _____   Hydrostatic pressure is greater than osmotic pressure

    _____   Net movement of fluid out of the capillary

    _____   Net movement of fluid into the capillary

3. In the spaces on the left, write the answers that match the statements about blood flow and blood pressure.

    _____   Vessel with the greatest pressure

    _____   Type of vessel with the greatest area

    _____   Type of vessel with the lowest pressure

    _____   Type of vessel with the slowest blood flow

    _____   Vessel with the fastest blood flow

_____ Primary force that moves blood

_____ Actions that move blood through veins (3)

_____

_____

_____ Pressure during ventricular contraction

_____ Pressure during ventricular relaxation

_____ Instrument used to measure blood pressure

_____ Systolic pressure minus diastolic pressure

_____ Blood flow sounds heard in a stethoscope

_____ Effect of increased CO_2 on precapillary sphincters

4. Identify the pulse points indicated on the following diagram.

A. _____

B. _____

C. _____

D. _____

E. _____

F. _____

G. _____

H. _____

5. In the spaces on the left, write the answers that match the statements about the regulation of blood pressure.

_____ Location of vasomotor and cardiac centers

_____ Center that regulates heart rate

_____ Center that regulates blood vessel diameter

_____ Type of receptors that respond when vessel walls stretch

_____ Type of receptors that respond to carbon dioxide and hydrogen ion concentrations

_____ Substance produced by the kidneys that has a role in blood pressure regulation

_____ Actions of angiotensin that increase blood pressure (2)

_____

_____ Hormone that conserves sodium ions to increase blood pressure

6. Place a check (√) in the appropriate column to indicate whether the given condition tends to increase or decrease blood pressure.

Given Condition	Increase	Decrease
A marked increase in blood volume		
An increase in heart rate		
Polycythemia		
Loss of body fluids		
Sympathetic stimulation of arterioles		
Vasodilation		
Production of angiotensin		
Slow heartbeat		

Circulatory Pathways

1. Fill in the blanks with the correct blood vessels and valves to complete the pathway of pulmonary circulation.

Right atrium → _____ → Right ventricle → _____ →

_____ → _____ → Capillaries of lungs →

_____ → Left atrium

2. Identify the arteries at the base of the brain as indicated on the following diagram.

   A. _____

   B. _____

   C. _____

   D. _____

   E. _____

   F. _____

   G. _____

3. In the space at the left, write the name of the artery that is described.

   _____   Branches from the ascending aorta

   _____   First, or most anterior, branch of aortic arch

   _____   Branch of the aortic arch to the left arm

   _____   Paired vessels that go to the brain (2)

   _____

   _____   Middle branch of the aortic arch

4. Name the major arteries described by each phrase.

   _____   Located in the arm

   _____   Located on the lateral side of the forearm

   _____   Located on the medial side of the forearm

   _____   Branch of celiac that supplies the liver

   _____   Branch of celiac that supplies the stomach

   _____   Supplies the pancreas and spleen

   _____   Supplies the small intestine and part of the colon

   _____   Paired vessels to the kidneys

   _____   Supplies the descending colon and rectum

   _____   Formed by bifurcation of the aorta

_____ Enters the pelvis and supplies the urinary bladder

_____ Located in the thigh region

_____ Located in the posterior knee region

_____ Supplies the posterior portion of the leg

_____ Supplies the anterior portion of the leg

5. Name the major veins described by each phrase.

_____ Large veins that enter the right atrium (2)

_____

_____ Join to form the superior vena cava

_____ Major vein from the brain

_____ Superficial vein on the medial side of the arm

_____ Superficial vein on the lateral side of the arm

_____ Vein at the elbow used for drawing blood

_____ Deep vein in the arm

_____ Drains the muscle tissue of the abdominal wall

_____ Vein from the liver that enters the inferior vena cava

_____ Vein that carries nutrient-rich blood to the liver

_____ Veins that form the hepatic portal vein (2)

_____

_____ Longest vein in the body

_____ Join to form the inferior vena cava

_____ Drains blood from the pelvic viscera

_____ Large deep vein in the thigh

_____ Drains the dorsal foot and anterior leg muscles

_____ Drains the posterior leg muscles

6. Name the feature of fetal circulation described by each phrase.

_____ Transports blood from the fetus to the placenta

_____ Transports blood from the placenta to the fetus

_____ Bypasses the liver

_____ Opening in the interatrial septum

_____   Shunt from the pulmonary trunk to the aorta

_____   Structure where gaseous exchange occurs

7. Follow the pathway for the flow of blood from the left ventricle to the right middle cerebral artery by filling in the blanks.

    Left ventricle → aortic semilunar valve → _____ → aortic arch →

    _____ → _____ → _____ → right middle

    cerebral artery.

8. Follow the pathway for the flow of blood from the left gonad (ovary or testicle) to the lateral side of the left forearm by filling in the blanks.

    Left gonad → left gonadal vein → _____ → _____ →

    _____ → _____ valve → _____ →

    _____ valve → _____ → _____ → capillaries

    of lungs → _____ → _____ → _____ valve

    → _____ → _____ valve → _____ →

    aortic arch → _____ → _____ → _____ →

    _____ → capillaries on lateral side of left forearm.

9. Follow the pathway for the flow of blood from the descending aorta to the capillaries of the spleen and then to the right atrium by filling in the blanks.

    Descending aorta → _____ → _____ → capillaries of the

    spleen → _____ → _____ → sinusoids of the liver →

    _____ → _____ → right atrium.

REVIEW QUESTIONS

1. If a pin penetrates an artery from the outside into the lumen, name the layers of the arterial wall, in sequence, through which it passes.

2. In what two ways are veins structurally different from arteries?

3. By what transport mechanism do oxygen and carbon dioxide move across the capillary wall?

4. What two pressures determine fluid movement across the capillary wall?

5. As blood flows from the aorta into the more numerous smaller vessels, what happens to the rate of flow?

6. Why does blood tend to pool, or accumulate, in the legs and feet when a person stands in one place for a long period?

7. What superficial artery in the wrist is used to take the pulse?

8. If you are given the information that the diastolic pressure is 78 mm Hg and the systolic pressure is 115 mm Hg, what is the pulse pressure?

9. When blood vessels lose their elasticity due to aging or atherosclerosis, what happens to blood pressure?

10. Suppose baroreceptors in the aortic arch detect a sudden increase in blood pressure and generate action potentials. What part of the brain receives these action potentials and how does it respond?

11. The kidneys secrete renin in response to decreases in blood pressure. By what mechanism does renin cause an increase in the blood pressure?

12. Through what two valves does the blood pass to get from the right atrium to the lungs to receive a new supply of oxygen?

13. What branch of the aortic arch supplies blood to the right arm and the right side of the head and neck?

14. What branch of the subclavian artery ascends the neck to supply blood to the brain?

15. What two vessels join to form the superior vena cava?

16. Trace the path of blood from the abdominal aorta to the spleen and back to the inferior vena cava.

17. What two features of the circulatory pathway in the fetus allow blood to bypass the immature lungs?

CHAPTER QUIZ

1. Which one of the following best describes the tunica media of arteries? (a) simple squamous epithelium; (b) smooth muscle; (c) connective tissue; (d) vasa vasorum; (e) adventitia

2. Which of the following does *not* describe veins? (a) they have thinner walls than arteries; (b) they have valves to prevent backflow; (c) the pressure in veins is lower than in arteries; (d) veins can hold more blood than arteries; (e) veins carry blood away from the heart.

3. Indicate whether each of the following will increase (I) or decrease (D) the rate of blood flow to a specific area.

   _____ Increase the blood pressure

   _____ Increase the resistance

   _____ Increase the cardiac output

   _____ Vasodilation

   _____ Increase in carbon dioxide concentration

   _____ Contraction of precapillary sphincters

   _____ Decrease in pH

4. Indicate whether each of the following refers to (A) systolic pressure; (B) diastolic pressure, or (C) pulse pressure. You may use the letters A, B, or C as indicated.

   _____ Pressure at which the first Korotkoff sound is heard

   _____ Normal is about 40 mm Hg

   _____ Blood begins to flow freely through the arteries

   _____ Normally is about 120 mm Hg

   _____ Normally is about 80 mm Hg

5. Assuming that other factors remain constant, what effect will each of the following have on blood pressure? I = Increase D = Decrease

   _____ Increase in heart rate

   _____ Decreased amounts of antidiuretic hormone (ADH)

   _____ Polycythemia

   _____ Decrease in blood volume

   _____ Vasodilation

   _____ Decreased elasticity in arterial walls

   _____ Stimulation of baroreceptors in the aortic arch

   _____ Epinephrine from adrenal medulla

   _____ Fluid retention

   _____ Increased angiotensin

6. Match the following descriptions with the appropriate artery. There is only one correct response for each description and not all responses will be used.

A. anterior tibial
B. brachiocephalic
C. celiac
D. common iliac
E. external iliac

F. femoral
G. hepatic
H. left common carotid
I. pulmonary
J. radial

K. renal
L. splenic
M. superior mesenteric
N. ulnar
O. vertebral

_____ Carries deoxygenated blood to the lungs

_____ Branch from the aortic arch that supplies the right arm, head, and neck

_____ Formed from the bifurcation of the abdominal aorta

_____ Branch of the subclavian artery that supplies blood to the brain

_____ Artery on the medial side of the forearm

_____ Branch of the abdominal aorta that supplies blood to the liver and spleen

_____ Branch of the abdominal aorta that supplies blood to most of the small intestine

_____ Large artery in the thigh

_____ Artery that supplies blood to the anterior portion of the leg

_____ Artery that supplies blood to the kidneys

7. Match the following descriptions with the appropriate vein. There is only one correct response for each description and not all responses will be used.

A. basilic
B. brachial
C. brachiocephalic
D. cephalic
E. common iliac
F. femoral

G. great saphenous
H. hepatic
I. hepatic portal
J. inferior vena cava
K. internal jugular

L. popliteal
M. radial
N. superior vena cava
O. ulnar
P. umbilical

_____ Receives blood from the venous sinuses of the brain

_____ Carries blood from the placenta to the fetal liver

_____ Receives blood from the head and upper extremities; empties into the right atrium

_____ Deep vein in the arm

_____ Single vein in the posterior knee region

_____ Superficial vein on the lateral side of the forearm and arm

_____ Drains blood from the liver into the inferior vena cava

_____ Superficial vein of the thigh and leg; drains into the femoral vein

_____ Vessel between the superior mesenteric vein and liver

_____ Veins that join to form the inferior vena cava

USING CLINICAL KNOWLEDGE

1. Match the definitions on the left with the correct term from the column on the right by placing the corresponding letter in the space before the definition. Not all terms will be used.

_____	Sounds heard in the stethoscope when taking blood pressure	A. Angioplasty
_____	Increase in size of the lumen of blood vessels	B. Arterectomy
_____	A calcium-channel blocker that may be used in the treatment of hypertension	C. Diltiazem hydrochloride
_____	Varicose veins in the anal canal	D. Furosemide
_____	Inflammation of veins	E. Hemangioma
_____	Opposition to blood flow	F. Hemorrhoids
_____	A diuretic used to decrease blood pressure	G. Ischemia
_____	Surgical repair of a blood vessel	H. Korotkoff
_____	A benign tumor of a blood vessel	I. Peripheral resistance
_____	Deficiency in blood supply due to constriction or obstruction of a vessel	J. Phlebitis
		K. Vasoconstriction
		L. Vasodilation

2. Write the meaning of the following abbreviations.

_____ CVP

_____ DSA

_____ KVO

_____ PTCA

_____ H&H

3. Spelling is important in scientific and medical applications because only one or two incorrect letters may change the meaning. All of the following words are from this chapter and are spelled incorrectly. Write the correct spelling in the space preceding the misspelled words.

_____ sfincters

_____ distolic

_____ sphygmanometer

_____ peracardial

_____ aneurism

4. Write the meaning of the underlined portion of each word on the line preceding the word.

_____ <u>athero</u>sclerosis

_____ <u>ischem</u>ia

_____ <u>brach</u>iocephalic

_____ arterio<u>ven</u>ous

_____ <u>vas</u>orum

_____ arterio<u>sten</u>osis

_____ athero<u>scler</u>osis

_____ brachio<u>cephal</u>ic

5. Use these word parts to write clinical terms that fit the given definitions.

angi-   dermat-   -itis   thrombo-
arter-   -ectomy   phleb-

_____ Inflammation of blood vessels in the skin

_____ Surgical excision of a vein

_____ Inflammation of any blood vessel

_____ Surgical excision of an artery

_____ Inflammation of a vein associated with clot formation

FUN AND GAMES

Find your way through this maze of letters by drawing a continuous line that traces the pathway of blood through the heart and pulmonary circulation. Start with the R at the arrow, draw a line to an adjacent I, then a G, and so on to complete right atrium. Continue through the heart and pulmonary circulation, including chambers, valves, vessels, and lungs, until you finish with the aorta. The consecutive letters of the words are always adjacent but may be in any direction. Do not use any letter more than one time and do not cross a line you have already drawn.

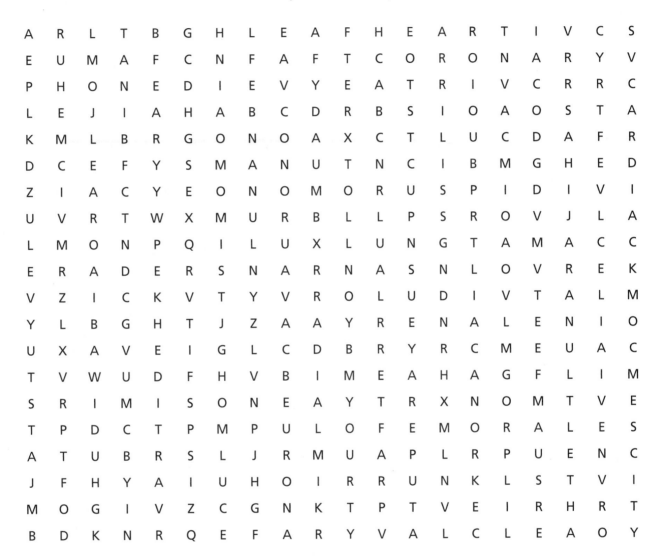

```
A  R  L  T  B  G  H  L  E  A  F  H  E  A  R  T  I  V  C  S
E  U  M  A  F  C  N  F  A  F  T  C  O  R  O  N  A  R  Y  V
P  H  O  N  E  D  I  E  V  Y  E  A  T  R  I  V  C  R  R  C
L  E  J  I  A  H  B  C  D  R  B  S  I  O  A  O  S  T  A
K  M  L  B  R  G  O  N  O  A  X  C  T  L  U  C  D  A  F  R
D  C  E  F  Y  S  M  A  N  U  T  N  C  I  B  M  G  H  E  D
Z  I  A  C  Y  E  O  N  O  M  O  R  U  S  P  I  D  I  V  I
U  V  R  T  W  X  M  U  R  B  L  L  P  S  R  O  V  J  L  A
L  M  O  N  P  Q  I  L  U  X  L  U  N  G  T  A  M  A  C  C
E  R  A  D  E  R  S  N  A  R  N  A  S  N  L  O  V  R  E  K
V  Z  I  C  K  V  T  Y  V  R  O  L  U  D  I  V  T  A  L  M
Y  L  B  G  H  T  J  Z  A  A  Y  R  E  N  A  L  E  N  I  O
U  X  A  V  E  I  G  L  C  D  B  R  Y  R  C  M  E  U  A  C
T  V  W  U  D  F  H  V  B  I  M  E  A  H  A  G  F  L  I  M
S  R  I  M  I  S  O  N  E  A  Y  T  R  X  N  O  M  T  V  E
T  P  D  C  T  P  M  P  U  L  O  F  E  M  O  R  A  L  E  S
A  T  U  B  R  S  L  J  R  M  U  A  P  L  R  P  U  E  N  C
J  F  H  Y  A  I  U  H  O  I  R  R  U  N  K  L  S  T  V  I
M  O  G  I  V  Z  C  G  N  K  T  P  T  V  E  I  R  H  R  T
B  D  K  N  R  Q  E  F  A  R  Y  V  A  L  C  L  E  A  O  Y
```

↑
Start

Lymphatic System and Body Defense

KEY TERMS

Active immunity
Antibody
Antigen
Artificial immunity
Immunoglobulin
Natural immunity
Passive immunity
Primary response
Resistance
Secondary response
Susceptibility

Anaphylaxis
Autoimmune disease
Immunologist
Interleukins
Kaposi's sarcoma
Lymphadenitis
Lymphangiogram
Lymphedema
Lymphoma
Metastasis
Mononucleosis
Oncologist
Splenomegaly

BUILDING VOCABULARY

aden-
-ectomy
immun-
lymph-
-lytic
-megaly
onc-
-pexy
splen-
thym-
-tic
tox-

CLINICAL ABBREVIATIONS

AIDS
CMV
DCIS
ELISA
HIV
HL
HZ
IDC
ILC
KS
NHL

CLINICAL TERMS

Acquired immunodeficiency syndrome
Allergen

OUTLINE/OBJECTIVES

Functions of the Lymphatic System

- State three functions of the lymphatic system.
  — The lymphatic system returns excess interstitial fluid to the blood.
  — The lymphatic system absorbs fats and fat-soluble vitamins from the digestive system.
  — The lymphatic system provides defense against invading microorganisms and disease.

Components of the Lymphatic System

- List the components of the lymphatic system, describe their structure, and explain their functions.
  — The lymphatic system consists of the lymph, lymphatic vessels, and lymphatic organs.
  — Lymphatic vessels carry fluid away from the tissues and return it to the venous system. The right lymphatic duct drains lymph from the upper right quadrant of the body. The thoracic duct, which begins in the abdomen as the cisterna chyli, drains the other 3/4 of the body. Lymphatic vessels have thin walls and have valves to prevent backflow of lymph.
  — Lymph nodes consist of dense masses of lymphocytes that are separated by spaces called lymph sinuses. Lymph enters a node through afferent vessels, filters through the sinuses, and leaves through an efferent vessel. Three areas in which lymph nodes tend to cluster are the inguinal nodes in the groin, axillary nodes in the armpit, and cervical nodes in the neck. There are no lymph nodes associated with the central nervous system. Lymph nodes filter and cleanse the lymph before it enters the blood.
  — Tonsils are clusters of lymphatic tissue in the region of the nose, mouth, and throat. They provide protection against pathogens that may enter through the nose and mouth. The pharyngeal tonsils, also called adenoids, are near the opening of the nasal cavity into the pharynx; palatine tonsils are near the opening of the oral cavity into the pharynx; and the lingual tonsils are at the base of the tongue, also near the opening of the oral cavity into the pharynx.
  — The spleen is located in the upper right quadrant of the abdomen, posterior to the stomach. It is much like a lymph node, but larger. It contains masses of lymphocytes and macrophages that are supported by a fibrous framework. The spleen filters blood in much the same way the lymph nodes filter lymph. The spleen also is a reservoir for blood.
  — The thymus is located anterior to the ascending aorta and posterior to the sternum. The principal function of the thymus is the processing and maturation of T-cells. It also produces thymosin that stimulates the maturation of lymphocytes in other organs.
- Describe the origin of lymph and describe the mechanisms that move the fluid through lymphatic vessels.
  — As soon as interstitial fluid enters lymphatic vessels, it is called lymph. Lymphatic vessels return lymph to the blood plasma.
  — Pressure gradients that move fluid through the lymphatic vessels come from skeletal muscle action, respiratory movements, and contraction of smooth muscle in vessel walls.

Resistance to Disease

- List four nonspecific mechanisms that provide resistance to disease and explain how each functions.
  — Disease-producing organisms are called pathogens. The ability to counteract pathogens is resistance, and a lack of resistance is susceptibility.
  — Nonspecific defense mechanisms include barriers, chemical action, phagocytosis, and inflammation.

— Barriers are factors that deter microbial invasion. They may be of a mechanical nature (unbroken skin), fluid (tears), or chemical (lysozymes).
— If microorganisms succeed in passing through the barriers, internal defenses, such as chemical action, respond. Complement is a chemical defense that promotes phagocytosis and inflammation. Interferon has particular significance because it offers protection against viruses. It is produced by virus-infected cells to provide protection for the neighboring cells.
— Phagocytosis is the ingestion and destruction of solid particles by certain cells, particularly neutrophils and macrophages. Neutrophils are small cells that are the first to migrate to an infected area. Macrophages are monocytes that leave the blood and enter the tissue spaces. They phagocytize cellular debris. They also perform a cleansing action on the lymph and blood.
— Inflammation is characterized by redness, warmth, swelling, and pain. Inflammation includes a series of events, outlined in Table 14-1 of the textbook, that occur in response to tissue damage. The overall purpose of inflammation is to destroy bacteria, cleanse the area of debris, and promote healing. Systemic inflammation is characterized by leukocytosis, fever, and a dangerous decrease in blood pressure.

- State the two characteristics of specific defense mechanisms and identify the two principal cells involved in specific resistance.
  — Specificity and memory are two features of specific defense mechanisms. The principal cells involved are lymphocytes and macrophages.
  — Proteins and other large molecules that are recognized as belonging to the body of an individual are interpreted as "self." Others are interpreted as "nonself." Antigens are molecules that trigger an immune response. Usually they are foreign proteins that enter the body and are interpreted as nonself.
  — During fetal development, the bone marrow releases immature lymphocytes into the blood. Some of the immature lymphocytes go to the thymus gland where they differentiate to become T-lymphocytes (T-cells). About 70% of the circulating lymphocytes are T-cells. Lymphocytes that differentiate in some region other than the thymus are B-lymphocytes (B-cells). These account for about 30% of the circulating lymphocytes.
- Briefly describe the mechanism of cell-mediated immunity and list four subgroups of T-cells.
  — Cell-mediated immunity is the result of T-cell action.
  — When an antigen enters the body, it is phagocytized by a macrophage, which presents the antigen to an appropriate T-cell. The T-cell responds by producing clones of T-cells.
  — Killer T-cells directly destroy the cells with the offending antigen; helper T-cells secrete substances that promote the immune response; suppressor T-cells inhibit the immune response and help regulate it; memory T-cells stimulate a faster and more intense response if the same antigen enters the body again.
- Briefly describe the mechanism of antibody-mediated immunity and list two subgroups of B-cells.
  — B-cells are responsible for antibody-mediated immunity.
  — When an antigen enters the body, a macrophage phagocytizes it and presents to the appropriate B-cell. The B-cell responds by forming clones of plasma cells and memory B-cells. Plasma cells produce large quantities of antibodies that inactivate the invading antigens.
- Distinguish between the primary response and the secondary response to a pathogen.
  — The initial action against a pathogen is a primary response.
  — If the same pathogen enters the body a second time, memory B-cells launch a rapid and intense response. This is called a secondary response, which is faster and more intense than the initial primary response.
- List five classes of immunoglobulins and state the role each has in immunity.
  — Antibodies belong to a class of proteins called globulins. Since they are involved in the immune response, they are called immunoglobulins.
  — IgA, IgG, IgM, IgE, and IgD are five classes of immunoglobulins. Each class has a specific role in immunity as indicated in Table 14-2 of the textbook.

- Give examples of active natural immunity, active artificial immunity, passive natural immunity, and passive artificial immunity.
  — Active immunity occurs when the body produces memory cells; passive immunity results when the immune agents are transferred into an individual. Natural immunity is acquired through normal activities; artificial requires some deliberate action.
  — Active natural immunity results when a person is exposed to a harmful antigen, contracts the disease, and recovers.
  — Active artificial immunity develops when a prepared antigen is deliberately introduced into the body (vaccination) and stimulates the immune system.
  — Passive natural immunity results when antibodies are transferred from mother to child through the placenta or milk.
  — Passive artificial immunity results when antibodies are injected into an individual.

LEARNING EXERCISES

Functions of the Lymphatic System

1. Three functions of the lymphatic system are to:

   (a)

   (b)

   (c)

Components of the Lymphatic System

1. Name the three major components of the lymphatic system.

   (a)

   (b)

   (c)

2. In the spaces on the left, write the answers that match the statements about lymph and lymphatic vessels.

   _____ Fluid within the tissue spaces

   _____ Source of fluid in tissue spaces

   _____ Fluid within lymphatic vessels

   _____ Source of fluid within lymphatic vessels

   _____ Smallest lymphatic vessels

   _____ Largest lymphatic vessels

   _____ Drains the upper right quadrant of the body

   _____ Collects lymph from 3/4 of the body

_____   Structure at beginning of thoracic duct

_____   Returns lymph to right subclavian vein

_____   Returns lymph to left subclavian vein

_____   Prevent backflow of lymph within vessels

_____   Actions that move lymph in vessels (3)

_____

_____

3. In the spaces on the left, write the answers that match the statements about the organs of the lymphatic system.

_____   Characteristic cells in lymphatic organs

_____   Located along lymphatic pathways

_____   Located near the mouth, nose, and throat

_____   Located posterior to the stomach

_____   Located near the heart

_____   Filters lymph

_____   Filters blood

_____   Protect against pathogens that enter via the nose

_____   Functions in maturation of T-lymphocytes

_____   Reservoir for blood

_____   Called adenoids when enlarged

_____   Carry lymph into a lymph node

_____   Hormone from the thymus

_____   Consists of red pulp and white pulp

Resistance to Disease

1. In the spaces on the left, write the words that are defined on the right.

_____   Disease-producing organisms

_____   Ability to counteract harmful agents

_____   Lack of resistance

_____   Mechanisms against all harmful agents

_____   Mechanisms against selected harmful agents

_____   Specific resistance

2. Systemic inflammation is a medical crisis. List three characteristics of systemic inflammation.

    (a)

    (b)

    (c)

3. Match each of the following processes, agents, and components with the nonspecific defense mechanism of which it is a part.

    A. barrier to entry
    B. protective chemical action
    C. phagocytosis
    D. inflammatory reaction

    _____ Unbroken skin and mucous membranes

    _____ Activates phagocytosis and inflammation

    _____ Blocks replication of viruses

    _____ Cilia action in the respiratory tract

    _____ Interferon

    _____ Accompanied by swelling, heat, and redness

    _____ Ingestion and destruction of solid particles by certain cells

    _____ Action of complement

    _____ Macrophages and neutrophils

    _____ Aimed at localizing damage and destroying its source

4. In the spaces on the left, write the answers that match the statements about specific defense mechanisms.

    _____ Characteristics of immunity (2)

    _____

    _____ Primary cell types involved in immunity (2)

    _____

    _____ Molecules that trigger immune responses

    _____ Lymphocytes that mature in the thymus

    _____ 30% of circulating lymphocytes

    _____ Responsible for cell-mediated immunity

    _____ Mature someplace other than in the thymus

    _____ Responsible for humoral immunity

_____   70% of circulating lymphocytes

_____   Produce antibodies

_____   Another term for antibodies

_____   Initial action against antigens

_____   Subgroups of T-cells (4)

_____

_____

_____

_____   Clones of B-cells (2)

_____

5. Write IgG, IgA, IgM, IgD, or IgE on the line preceding each phrase to identify the class of antibodies it describes.

_____   Most numerous antibody

_____   Responsible for allergic reactions

_____   Found in breast milk, saliva, mucus, and tears

_____   Responsible for ABO transfusion reactions

_____   Major antibody in immune responses

_____   Binds to mast cells and causes release of histamine

_____   Crosses placenta to provide immunity for newborn

_____   Causes agglutination of antigens

6. Match each of the following descriptions with the type of immunity it characterizes.

A. active natural   B. active artificial
C. passive natural   D. passive artificial

_____   Antiserum is injected into an individual

_____   A person contracts a disease, recovers, and is immune to that disease

_____   Antibodies are transferred from one person to another through natural processes

_____   Antigens deliberately introduced into a person to stimulate immunity

_____   Memory cells produced after contracting a disease such as chickenpox

_____   Antibodies injected into an individual after a poisonous snakebite

_____   IgA antibodies in mother's milk may provide some immunity for infants

_____   Mumps, diphtheria, whooping cough, and tetanus vaccines

REVIEW QUESTIONS

1. What are the three primary functions of the lymphatic system?

2. What three basic components make up the lymphatic system?

3. What is lymph?

4. What part of the body is drained by the thoracic duct? What part is drained by the right lymphatic duct?

5. Since there is no pump to move fluid through the lymphatic vessels, what provides the pressure gradients that are necessary to move the lymph?

6. For what purpose and by what pathway does lymph flow through lymph nodes?

7. What is the purpose of tonsils and where are they located?

8. What structural feature of the spleen characterizes it as a lymphatic organ? List two functions of the spleen.

9. When is the thymus most active and what is its function?

10. Use the term pathogen in a definition of resistance.

11. What is meant when a defense mechanism is said to be nonspecific? Give an example.

12. Give an example of a mechanical barrier that inhibits the entry of pathogens.

13. What is the particular significance of interferon in body defense?

14. What is the role of neutrophils and macrophages in body defense?

15. What are the four characteristics of localized inflammation? What are three additional characteristics of systemic inflammation?

16. In addition to their specificity, what is another feature of specific defense mechanisms?

17. What is an antigen?

18. What percentage of the circulating lymphocytes are normally T-cells? Where do they differentiate into T-cells?

19. What four clones of cells are produced in cell-mediated immunity?

20. What is the function of plasma cells and with what specific type of immunity are they associated?

21. In antibody-mediated immunity, which is more rapid—the primary response or the secondary response?

22. What is the meaning of the abbreviation Ig?

23. Which type of immunoglobulin is most numerous in blood plasma?

24. What is the source of antibodies in passive immunity?

25. An individual receives a vaccination that contains a specially prepared antigen. What type of immunity is acquired through this procedure?

CHAPTER QUIZ

1. The lymphatic vessel that drains lymph from the entire body *except* the upper right quadrant is the (a) right lymphatic duct; (b) lacteal; (c) cisterna chyli; (d) thoracic duct.

2. The *primary* function of lymph nodes is to (a) filter and cleanse the blood; (b) produce lymphocytes; (c) filter and cleanse lymph; (d) act as a reservoir for lymph.

3. Which of the following is *not* a function of the spleen? (a) filter and cleanse blood; (b) produce lymphocytes; (c) act as a reservoir for blood; (d) filter and cleanse lymph

4. T-lymphocytes differentiate in the _____.

5. Match each of the following with the nonspecific defense mechanism with which it is most closely associated.

   _____ Intact skin   A. barriers

   _____ Interferon and complement   B. phagocytosis

   _____ Lysozymes in tears   C. chemicals

   _____ Swelling and pain   D. inflammation

   _____ Neutrophils and macrophages

   _____ Fluid flow (urine)

6. The primary cells involved in specific resistance are _____ and _____.

7. Indicate whether each of the following refers to T-cells, B-cells, or both T- and B-cells.

   T = T-cells   B = B-cells   TB = both

   _____ Memory cells

   _____ Cell-mediated immunity

   _____ Plasma cells

   _____ Humoral immunity

   _____ Antibodies

   _____ Clones of helper and killer cells

   _____ Macrophage presents antigen

   _____ Immunoglobulins

8. The type of immunity acquired by obtaining a vaccination that consists of a weakened pathogen is (a) active natural immunity; (b) active artificial immunity; (c) passive natural immunity; (d) passive artificial immunity.

USING CLINICAL KNOWLEDGE

1. Match the definitions on the left with the correct term from the column on the right by placing the corresponding letter in the space before the definition. Not all terms will be used.

_____	A substance that triggers an immune response	A. Anaphylaxis
_____	Immunity produced when antibodies are passed through breast milk from mother to infant	B. Antibody
		C. Antigen
_____	Used to reduce rejection of kidney and liver transplants	D. Antisera
		E. Artificial
_____	Specialist in the diagnosis and treatment of malignant disorders	F. Immunosuppressants
		G. Lymphoma
_____	Malignant tumor of lymph nodes/lymph tissue	H. Metastasis
_____	Ability to counteract the effects of pathogens	I. Oncologist
_____	Detoxified antigenic agents that induce antibody formation	J. Passive
		K. Resistance
_____	An exaggerated or unusual hypersensitivity reaction to a foreign protein	L. Splenomegaly
_____	Spread of a tumor to a secondary site	M. Susceptibility
_____	Enlargement of the spleen	N. Toxoids

2. Write the meaning of the following abbreviations.

    _____ AIDS

    _____ CMV

    _____ KS

    _____ HIV

    _____ IDC

3. Spelling is important in scientific and medical applications because only one or two incorrect letters may change the meaning. All of the following words are from this chapter, but only two are spelled incorrectly. Place a check (√) in the space preceding the words that are spelled correctly. Write the correct spelling in the space preceding the misspelled words.

    _____ immunoglobulins

    _____ eferent

    _____ vaccination

    _____ pyrogens

    _____ thorasic

4. Write the meaning of the underlined portion of each word on the line preceding the word.

_____ to<u>x</u>oid

_____ <u>immun</u>ology

_____ hemo<u>lytic</u>

_____ <u>onc</u>ology

_____ <u>lymphangi</u>ography

5. Separate the following words into their component parts, give the definition of each part, then put the parts together to write a definition for the entire word.

lymphadenopathy _____

_____

_____

splenorrhagia _____

_____

_____

6. Mary Lynn Fatic was diagnosed with breast cancer and had a portion of the breast tissue removed. During the procedure, the surgeon also excised the axillary lymph nodes. After the surgery, she developed swelling in her arm.

   a. Why were the lymph nodes removed?

   b. What caused the swelling in the arm?

   c. What is the medical term for the swelling she experienced?

FUN AND GAMES

Fill in the blanks by answering the clues at the bottom of the page.

1. — — — — **I** — — —

2. — — — **M** — —

3. — — **M** — — — — — — — —

4. — — — **U** — — — — — — — — — —

5. — **N** — — — — — — — —

6. — — — — **O** — — — — —

7. — — — — — **L** — — —

8. — — — — — **O** — — — —

9. — — — — **G** — —

10. — **Y** — — — — — —

11. — — **A** — — — — — —

12. — **N** — — — — — — — —

13. — — **T** — — — — — —

14. — — — — **I** — — — — —

15. — — **B** — —

16. — — — — **O** — — — — — —

17. — — — — — — **D** — — — — —

18. — — — **I** — —

19. — — — — — **E** — —

20. — — **S** — — — — — — — — — — —

Clues

1. Lymphoid tissue in pharynx
2. Processes certain lymphocytes
3. WBC involved in immunity
4. Another name for antibodies
5. Protein that stimulates T-cells
6. Large phagocytic cell
7. Exaggerated hypersensitivity response
8. Small phagocytic cell
9. Non-self molecule
10. Enzyme in tears and saliva
11. Produces antibodies
12. Mechanical barrier against pathogens
13. Inhibits viral replication
14. Injection of inactivated pathogens
15. Sign of inflammation
16. Cellular ingestion of pathogens
17. Inflammation of lymph glands
18. Type of immunity
19. Cause fever
20. Opposite of resistance

15

Respiratory System

KEY TERMS

Alveolus
Bronchial tree
Bronchopulmonary segment
External respiration
Internal respiration
Respiratory membrane
Surfactant
Ventilation

BUILDING VOCABULARY

-a
alveol-
anthrac-
atel-
bronchi-
-capnia
-coni-
cric-
dys-
-ectasis
eu-
laryng-
-ole
phon-
phren-
-pnea
pneum-
-ptysis
pulmon-
rhin-
-rrhea
spir-
thyr-
-tion
ventilat-

CLINICAL TERMS

Aspiration
Atelectasis
Bronchogenic carcinoma
Chronic obstructive pulmonary disease (COPD)
Coryza
Croup
Hemoptysis
Pertussis
Phrenitis
Pneumoconiosis
Pneumonectomy
Pneumothorax
Pulmonary edema
Rhinoplasty
Smoker's respiratory syndrome
Thoracocentesis

CLINICAL ABBREVIATIONS

CF
COPD
CRD
IPF
IPPB
PEEP
PFT
RDS
SAS
SIDS
SOB
SRS
TB
URI
VC

OUTLINE/OBJECTIVES

Functions and Overview of Respiration

- Define five activities of the respiratory process.
  — The entire process of respiration includes ventilation, external respiration, transport of gases, internal respiration, and cellular respiration.

Ventilation

- Describe the structures and features of the upper respiratory tract and the lower respiratory tract.
  — The upper respiratory tract includes the nose, pharynx, and larynx. The lower respiratory tract consists of the trachea, bronchial tree, and lungs.
  — The nasal cavity opens to the outside through the external nares and into the pharynx through the internal nares. It is separated from the oral cavity by the palate. The frontal, maxillary, ethmoidal, and sphenoidal sinuses are air-filled cavities that open into the nasal cavity. Air is warmed, moistened, and filtered as it passes through the nasal cavity.
  — The region of the pharynx is divided into the nasopharynx, oropharynx, and the laryngopharynx. Pharyngeal tonsils are located in the wall of the nasopharynx, but the palatine and lingual tonsils are located in the oropharynx. The auditory tubes open into the nasopharynx. The opening from the oral cavity into the oropharynx is the fauces.
  — The larynx is formed by nine cartilages that are connected to each other by muscles and ligaments. The three largest cartilages are the thyroid, cricoid, and epiglottis. There are two pairs of folds in the larynx. The upper pair are the vestibular folds. The lower pair are the true vocal cords. The opening between the vocal cords is the glottis.
  — The framework of the trachea is supported by 15 to 20 C-shaped pieces of hyaline cartilage. The mucous membrane that lines the trachea has goblet cells and cilia. The goblet cells secrete mucus that traps inhaled particles, and the cilia provide a cleansing action to remove the mucus with the particles.
  — The trachea divides into the right and left primary bronchi, which then divide into secondary (lobar) bronchi, and these into tertiary (segmental) bronchi. The branching pattern continues into smaller and smaller passageways until they terminate in tiny air sacs called alveoli.
- Describe the structure of the lungs including shape, lobes, tissue, and membranes.
  — The right lung is shorter, broader, and has a greater volume than the left lung.
  — The right lung is divided into 3 lobes; the left lung has 2 lobes.
  — The left lung has an indentation, called the cardiac notch, for the apex of the heart.
  — The lungs consist of the bronchial tree, except for the primary bronchi, which are outside the lungs. The alveoli of the lungs consist of simple squamous epithelium, which permits rapid diffusion of oxygen and carbon dioxide.
  — The parietal pleura lines the wall of the thorax; the visceral pleura is firmly attached to the surface of the lung. The pleural cavity is the space between the two layers of pleura.
- Name and define three pressures involved in pulmonary ventilation and relate these pressures to the sequence of events that results in inspiration and expiration.
  — Air flows because of pressure differences between the atmosphere and the gases inside the lungs. Atmospheric pressure is the pressure of the air outside the body. Intraalveolar (intrapulmonary) pressure is the pressure inside the alveoli of the lungs. Intrapleural pressure is the pressure within the pleural cavity, the space between the visceral and parietal pleurae.
  — During inspiration the diaphragm contracts and the thoracic cavity increases in volume. An increase in thoracic volume decreases the pressure below atmospheric pressure so that air flows into the lungs.
  — During expiration, the relaxation of the diaphragm and elastic recoil of tissues decrease the thoracic volume. The decrease in thoracic volume increases the intraalveolar pressure so that

air flows out of the lungs. Surfactant reduces the surface tension inside the alveoli so they do not adhere to each other and collapse.

- Define four respiratory volumes and four respiratory capacities. State their average normal values for an adult male, and describe factors that influence them.
  - The four respiratory volumes measured by spirometry are tidal volume (500 ml), inspiratory reserve volume (3100 ml), expiratory reserve volume (1200 ml), and residual volume (1200 ml).
  - A respiratory capacity is the sum of two or more volumes. Four respiratory capacities are the vital capacity (4800 ml), inspiratory capacity (3600 ml), functional residual capacity (2400 ml), and total lung capacity (6000 ml).
  - Age, sex, body build, and physical conditioning have an influence on lung volumes and capacities.

Basic Gas Laws and Respiration

- Discuss factors that govern the diffusion of gases into and out of the blood.
  - Dalton's law of partial pressures states that the total pressure exerted by a mixture of gases is equal to the sum of the pressures exerted by each gas independently, and the partial pressure exerted by each gas is proportional to its percentage in the total mixture.
  - Henry's law states that when a mixture of gases is in contact with a liquid, each gas dissolves in the liquid in proportion to its own solubility and partial pressure.
- Distinguish between external respiration and internal respiration.
  - External respiration is the exchange of gases between the lungs and the pulmonary capillaries. The surfaces in the lungs where diffusion occurs are called the respiratory membranes. The layers of the respiratory membrane are the (1) thin layer of fluid that lines the alveolus, (2) simple squamous epithelium in the alveolar wall, (3) basement membrane of the epithelium, (4) small interstitial space, (5) basement membrane of capillary epithelium, and (6) simple squamous epithelium of the capillary wall.
  - The rate at which external respiration occurs varies with the surface area and thickness of the respiratory membrane, the solubility of the gas, and the difference in partial pressure of the gas on the two sides of the membrane.
  - Internal respiration is the exchange of gases between the tissue cells and the blood in the tissue capillaries. Oxygen diffuses from the blood into the tissue cells and carbon dioxide diffuses from the tissue cells into the blood.

Transport of Gases

- Describe how oxygen and carbon dioxide are transported in the blood.
  - Approximately 3% of the oxygen is transported as a dissolved gas in the plasma. The remaining 97% is carried by hemoglobin molecules as oxyhemoglobin. Loading occurs in the lungs when oxygen combines with hemoglobin. It takes place when oxygen levels are high and carbon dioxide levels are low. Unloading occurs in the tissues when hemoglobin releases oxygen. It occurs when oxygen levels are low, carbon dioxide levels are high, temperature is increased, and pH is decreased.
  - Approximately 7% of the carbon dioxide is transported as a gas dissolved in the plasma. Another 23% of the carbon dioxide combines with the protein portion of hemoglobin and is transported as carbaminohemoglobin. The remaining 70% of the carbon dioxide is transported as bicarbonate ions in the plasma.
  - In the lungs, where carbon dioxide levels are relatively low, reactions occur that release the carbon dioxide from its transport forms. The carbon dioxide diffuses into the alveoli and is exhaled.

Regulation of Respiration

- Name two regions in the brain that make up the respiratory center and two nerves that carry impulses from the center.
  - The respiratory center includes groups of inspiratory and expiratory neurons in the medulla oblongata and pons.
  - The inspiratory area sends impulses along the phrenic nerve to the diaphragm and along the intercostal nerves to the external intercostal muscles. When inspiratory impulses cease, the muscles relax, and expiration occurs. When more forceful expiration is necessary, the expiratory center sends impulses along the intercostal nerves to the internal intercostal muscles.
- Describe the role of chemoreceptors, stretch receptors, higher brain centers, and temperature in regulating breathing.
  - Central chemoreceptors in the medulla oblongata are sensitive to increases in carbon dioxide and hydrogen ion levels. Peripheral chemoreceptors in the aortic and carotid bodies detect decreases in oxygen levels, but this is not a strong stimulus for breathing.
  - Stretch receptors in the lungs initiate the Hering-Breuer reflex that prevents overinflation of the lungs.
  - Voluntary or involuntary impulses from the higher brain centers may override the respiratory center temporarily, but after a limited time the respiratory center resumes control.
  - An increase in temperature increases the breathing rate.

LEARNING EXERCISES

Functions and Overview of Respiration

1. In the spaces on the left, write the terms that match the phrases about the sequence of events in respiration.

   _____ Exchange of air between atmosphere and lungs

   _____ Exchange of gases between lungs and blood

   _____ Function of blood in respiration

   _____ Exchange of gases between blood and tissues

   _____ Utilization of oxygen in the cells

Ventilation

1. Use the letter U to designate the regions of the upper respiratory tract and the letter L to designate the regions of the lower respiratory tract.

   _____ Bronchi   _____ Pharynx

   _____ Nose   _____ Lungs

   _____ Larynx   _____ Trachea

2. In the spaces on the left, write the answers that match the phrases about the respiratory tract.

_____ Functions of the nasal cavity (3)

_____

_____

_____ Region of pharynx posterior to the nasal cavity

_____ Location of the pharyngeal tonsils

_____ Pharynx from the uvula to the hyoid bone

_____ Lowest region of the pharynx

_____ Cartilage that forms the Adam's apple

_____ Most inferior cartilage of the larynx

_____ Prevents food from entering the larynx

_____ Opening between the true vocal cords

_____ Passage commonly called the windpipe

_____ Ridge of cartilage at bifurcation of the trachea

_____ Tissue that forms lining of the trachea

_____ Tissue that forms the alveoli

3. Arrange the following air passages in the correct sequence from largest to smallest by placing the numbers 1 to 7 in the spaces before the names. Use number 1 for the largest and number 7 for the smallest.

_____ Alveolar ducts   _____ Lobar bronchi

_____ Respiratory bronchioles   _____ Terminal bronchioles

_____ Alveoli   _____ Primary bronchi

_____ Segmental bronchi

4. Place an R in the space preceding the phrase if it refers to the right lung. Place an L in the space if it refers to the left lung. If the phrase applies to both lungs, place a B in the space.

_____ Cardiac notch   _____ Rests on the diaphragm

_____ Two lobes   _____ Has two fissures

_____ Shorter and wider   _____ Enclosed by the pleura

_____ Divided into lobules   _____ Anchored at the root or hilum

5. In the spaces on the left, write the answers that match the phrases about pulmonary ventilation.

_____ Name of pressure between layers of pleurae

_____ Name of pressure outside the body

_____ Name of pressure within the alveoli

_____ Pressure that is normally less than the two others

_____ Primary muscle involved in quiet breathing

_____ Muscles used in forced expiration

_____ Reduces surface tension within the alveoli

_____ Instrument to measure respiratory volumes

_____ Highest pressure during expiration

_____ Highest pressure during inspiration

6. Write I in the space if the event occurs during inspiration, and write E if it occurs during expiration.

_____ Diaphragm contracts

_____ Intrapulmonary pressure exceeds atmospheric pressure

_____ External intercostal muscles may contract

_____ Atmospheric pressure is greater than intrapulmonary pressure

_____ Lung volume increases

_____ Diaphragm relaxes

_____ Internal intercostal muscles may contract

_____ Air flows into the lungs

_____ Elastic recoil decreases the size of the alveoli

7. Match the lung volumes and capacities with their definitions.

TV = Tidal volume   VC = Vital capacity
IRV = Inspiratory reserve volume   IC = Inspiratory capacity
ERV = Expiratory reserve volume   FRC = Functional residual capacity
RV = Residual volume   TLC = Total lung capacity

_____ Maximum amount of air that can be inhaled

_____ Amount of air inhaled and exhaled in a quiet breathing cycle

_____ Amount of air in lungs after quiet expiration

_____ Equals TV + IRV + ERV

_____ Maximum amount of air that can be inhaled after a tidal inspiration

_____ Amount of air in lungs after maximum inspiration

_____ Maximum amount of air that can be forcefully exhaled after tidal expiration

_____ Equals RV + ERV

_____ Amount of air in lungs after maximum expiration

_____ Equals RV + ERV + TV + IRV

8. Complete the following table by writing in the correct values in the blank spaces.

TLC	VC	TV	ERV	IRV	RV
		500 ml	1000 ml	3000 ml	1200 ml
6000 ml	5000 ml		900 ml	3500 ml	
	4700 ml	600 ml	800 ml		1100 ml
5900 ml	4600 ml	400 ml		3000 ml	

9. If the individual type on the left tends to have greater lung volume than the type on the right, write > (greater than) on the blank in the center. If the left type tends to have less lung volume than the type on the right, write < (less than).

Young adults	_____	Senior citizens
Females	_____	Males
Short people	_____	Tall people
Normal weight people	_____	Obese people
Healthy people	_____	People with muscular disease
Good physical condition	_____	Poor physical condition

Basic Gas Laws and Respiration

1. Atmospheric air is a mixture of oxygen, nitrogen, and carbon dioxide. According to Dalton's law of partial pressures, if the atmospheric pressure is 750 mm Hg and the oxygen content is 21%, what is the pressure due to oxygen?

2. According to Henry's law, what two factors determine how much of each gas in a mixture will dissolve in a liquid?

3. Complete the following statements that define external and internal respiration.

   External respiration is the exchange of gases between the _____ and the _____.

   Internal respiration is the exchange of gases between the _____ and the _____.

4. List, in sequence, the six layers of the respiratory membrane through which oxygen must pass to diffuse from the alveolus into the blood capillary.

(a)   (d)

(b)   (e)

(c)   (f)

5. Indicate whether each of the following will increase or decrease the rate of gaseous exchange across the respiratory membrane. Use I for increase and D for decrease.

_____ Decreasing the surface area of the respiratory membrane

_____ Fluid accumulation in the alveoli due to pulmonary edema

_____ Increasing tidal volume

_____ Decreasing breathing rate

Transport of Gases

1. List two ways in which oxygen is transported in the blood.

(a)

(b)

2. List three ways in which carbon dioxide is transported in the blood.

(a)

(b)

(c)

3. In the spaces on the left, write the answers that match the phrases about oxygen and carbon dioxide transport.

_____   Compound in which most oxygen is transported

_____   Method of most carbon dioxide transport

_____   Combination of carbon dioxide and hemoglobin

_____   Combination of water and carbon dioxide

_____   Enzyme that speeds up the reaction between water and carbon dioxide

4. Place a check (√) in front of the factors in the tissues that favor unloading of oxygen.

_____ Increased partial pressure of oxygen

_____ Increased partial pressure of carbon dioxide

_____ Increased hydrogen ion concentration

_____ Increased temperature

_____ Increased pH

_____ Increased cellular metabolism

5. Place an E before the phrases that refer to external respiration, and place an I before the phrases that refer to internal respiration.

_____ Oxygen diffuses into the blood

_____ Oxygen diffuses out of the blood

_____ Carbon dioxide diffuses into the blood

_____ Carbon dioxide diffuses out of the blood

_____ Occurs in the alveolus

_____ Occurs in the body tissues

_____ Bicarbonate ion is formed

_____ Bicarbonate ions release carbon dioxide

_____ Oxyhemoglobin is formed

_____ Oxyhemoglobin dissociates and releases oxygen

Regulation of Respiration

1. The respiratory center includes neurons in the _____ and
_____.

2. The inspiratory areas of the respiratory center send impulses along the _____ nerve to the diaphragm and along the _____ nerves to the external intercostal muscles.

3. Place a T before each true statement and an F before each false statement about factors that influence the rate and depth of breathing.

_____ Chemoreceptors in the medulla oblongata are sensitive to changes in oxygen levels.

_____ Increases in blood CO_2 levels increase the rate and depth of breathing.

_____ Increases in hydrogen ion concentrations increase the rate and depth of breathing.

_____ Chemoreceptors in the medulla oblongata are sensitive to changes in carbon dioxide and hydrogen ion concentrations.

_____ A decrease in oxygen levels is usually a strong stimulus for breathing.

_____ Decreased oxygen levels usually make the respiratory center more sensitive to carbon dioxide changes.

_____ Peripheral chemoreceptors are located in the aortic and carotid bodies.

_____ The Hering-Breuer reflex prevents overinflation of the lungs.

_____ The Hering-Breuer reflex is a response to stretch receptors in the lungs.

_____ Higher brain centers may permanently override the respiratory center.

_____ Anxiety decreases the rate and depth of breathing.

_____ Chronic pain stimulates breathing, but sudden pain may cause a momentary cessation of breathing.

_____ Decreasing body temperature increases the breathing rate.

_____ The primary stimulus for breathing is decreased carbon dioxide levels in the respiratory center.

REVIEW QUESTIONS

1. List the five activities of the total respiratory process.

2. What structures are in the upper respiratory tract? Which ones are in the lower respiratory tract?

3. What are the external nares, internal nares, hard palate, soft palate, uvula, and nasal conchae?

4. What are the functions of the nasal cavity?

5. In what specific regions of the pharynx are the pharyngeal, palatine, and lingual tonsils located?

6. What are the three largest cartilages in the larynx?

7. What type of cartilage forms the framework of the trachea?

8. What two structural features of the tracheal lining function to prevent dirt and other particles from entering the lower respiratory tract?

9. Trace the branching of the bronchial tree from the trachea to the alveoli in the lungs.

10. What structural feature of the alveoli permits the rapid diffusion of gases?

11. How many lobes are in the right lung? Left lung?

12. What is between the parietal pleura and the visceral pleura?

13. During inspiration, which one of the three pressures involved in pulmonary ventilation is the greatest?

14. Why is inspiration considered an active process while expiration is a passive process?

15. What substance reduces surface tension within the alveoli?

16. Identify four respiratory volumes and four respiratory capacities on a spirogram.

17. How do age, sex, body build, and physical conditioning affect lung volumes and capacities?

18. What two properties of gases (gas laws) have an effect on the diffusion of a gas?

19. A molecule of oxygen diffuses from the alveolus to capillary blood during external respiration. Name, in sequence, the six layers it must pass through.

20. If the thickness of the respiratory membrane increases and other factors remain constant, how is the rate of external respiration affected?

21. Where does internal respiration take place?

22. How does an increase in carbon dioxide concentration affect the ability of oxygen to combine with hemoglobin?

23. Which normally provides more stimulus for breathing—a decrease in oxygen or an increase in carbon dioxide?

24. How is most of the carbon dioxide transported by the blood?

25. Where is the respiratory center located in the brain?

26. What nerve sends inspiratory impulses to the diaphragm? To the external intercostal muscles?

CHAPTER QUIZ

1. The pathway of inhaled air is
   (a) nasal cavity, trachea, larynx, bronchi, pharynx, alveoli
   (b) nasal cavity, pharynx, larynx, trachea, bronchi, alveoli
   (c) nasal cavity, larynx, pharynx, trachea, bronchi, alveoli
   (d) nasal cavity, pharynx, trachea, bronchi, larynx, alveoli
   (e) nasal cavity, pharynx, trachea, larynx, bronchi, alveoli

2. The following pairs of terms indicate a region of the pharynx and a structure or opening located in that region. Which pair is mismatched?
   (a) nasopharynx/openings for auditory tubes
   (b) oropharynx/fauces
   (c) oropharynx/palatine tonsils
   (d) laryngopharynx/pharyngeal tonsils
   (e) nasopharynx/adenoids

3. The following statements are about the lungs and pleura. Place a T before the true statements and an F before the false statements.

   _____ The left lung has three lobes and is longer than the right lung.

   _____ The pleural cavity is between the visceral pleura and the alveoli.

   _____ The heart makes an indentation, called the cardiac notch, in the left lung.

   _____ The lungs are divided into bronchopulmonary segments, each with its own segmental bronchus.

4. Given atmospheric pressure that 760 mm Hg, intraalveolar pressure that 763 mm Hg, and intrapleural pressure that 756 mm Hg, which of the following is indicated?
   (a) inspiration phase of ventilation
   (b) expiration phase of ventilation
   (c) period after expiration but before the next inspiration

5. Given that for a particular patient the tidal volume = 450 ml, inspiratory reserve volume = 2800 ml, expiratory reserve volume = 1050 ml, and residual volume = 1200 ml, what is this patient's vital capacity?
   (a) 1500 ml
   (b) 3250 ml
   (c) 5500 ml
   (d) 4300 ml
   (e) 3850 ml

6. Which of the following is *not* true about external respiration?
   (a) Carbon dioxide enters the blood and oxygen enters the alveoli.
   (b) Gases diffuse across the respiratory membrane in the lungs.
   (c) An accumulation of fluid in the alveoli decreases the diffusion rate.
   (d) Surface area of the alveoli affects the diffusion rate.

7. The affinity of hemoglobin and oxygen decreases when
   (a) hydrogen ion concentration decreases
   (b) carbon dioxide levels increase
   (c) temperature decreases
   (d) oxygen levels increase

8. More than 2/3 of the carbon dioxide transported in the blood is
   (a) dissolved in the plasma
   (b) bound to hemoglobin
   (c) attached to carbonic anhydrase
   (d) in the form of bicarbonate ions

9. The respiratory center in the brain includes neurons in the
   (a) cerebrum and cerebellum
   (b) thalamus and pons
   (c) midbrain and medulla oblongata
   (d) medulla oblongata and pons

10. Chemoreceptors in the central nervous system stimulate inspiration when they detect
    (a) low oxygen levels
    (b) low hydrogen ion and high carbon dioxide levels
    (c) increased hydrogen ion and carbon dioxide levels
    (d) increased hydrogen ion and decreased carbon dioxide levels

USING CLINICAL KNOWLEDGE

1. Match the definitions on the left with the correct term from the column on the right by placing the corresponding letter in the space before the definition. Not all terms will be used.

_____	Movement of air into and out of the lungs	A. Antitussives
_____	Inflammation of the diaphragm	B. Atelectasis
_____	Accumulation of air in the pleural space	C. Coryza
_____	Whooping cough	D. External respiration
_____	Suppress the cough reflex in the medulla oblongata	E. Hemoptysis
_____	Exchange of gases between the lungs and blood	F. Internal respiration
_____	Spitting of blood from bleeding in the respiratory tract	G. Mucolytics
_____	Common cold	H. Pertussis
_____	Swelling and fluid in the alveoli and bronchioles	I. Phrenitis
_____	Break down mucus and promote coughing	J. Pneumothorax
		K. Pulmonary edema
		L. Ventilation

2. Write the meaning of the following abbreviations.

_____ VC

_____ CRD

_____ IPPB

_____ RDS

_____ SRS

3. Spelling is important in scientific and medical applications because only one or two incorrect letters may change the meaning. Circle the correctly spelled word for each of the following pairs.

intraalveolar	intralveolar
diaphram	diaphragm
larynx	larnyx
pleura	plura
emphysemia	emphysema

4. Write the meaning of the underlined portion of each word on the line preceding the word.

_____ pneumo<u>coni</u>osis

_____ hyper<u>capni</u>a

_____ <u>rhino</u>plasty

_____   atel<u>ectas</u>is

_____   dys<u>pnea</u>

_____   hemo<u>ptysis</u>

_____   dys<u>phon</u>ia

_____   rhino<u>rrhea</u>

_____   bronchi<u>ole</u>

_____   <u>anthrac</u>osis

5. Russ P. Tory worked in an environment with high levels of dust pollution. After several years, he developed shortness of breath, chronic cough, and expectoration of mucus containing particles of dust. His condition forced him to quit his job. What is the medical word for this group of lung diseases?

FUN AND GAMES

Each of the following clues is preceded by a plus (+) or minus (−) sign. Answer each clue. The number in parentheses indicates the number of letters in the answer to the clue. If there is a plus (+) preceding the clue, add the letters of your answer to the letters from previous answers. If there is a minus (−) preceding the clue, remove the letters of your answer from the previous letters. When you finish, there should be one letter remaining.

Example:

+ 1. A feline (3) CAT
    Letters: CAT

+ 2. A rodent (3) RAT
    Letters: CATRAT

− 3. A type of wagon (4) CART
    Letters: AT

− 4. First letter of the alphabet (1) A
    Letters: T

The final letter remaining is T. T is for TIME. It is TIME now for Fun and Games.

Clues

+ 1. Throat (7)
    Letters:

+ 2. Membrane around lungs (6)
    Letters:

− 3. Voice box (6)
    Letters:

+ 4. Reduces surface tension (10)
    Letters:

+ 5. Root for mouth or opening (2)
    Letters:

− 6. Cessation of breathing (5)
    Letters:

+ 7. Nostrils (5)
    Letters:

− 8. Opening from mouth into pharynx (6)
    Letters:

− 9. Prefix for lacking or without (1)
    Letters:

+ 10. Bifurcation of trachea (6)
    Letters:

Clues

+ 11. Air sac in lungs (8)
    Letters:

− 12. Swiss mountain (3)
    Letters:

− 13. Continues after larynx (7)
    Letters:

+ 14. Lung collapse (11)
    Letters:

+ 15. Major respiratory muscle (9)
    Letters:

− 16. What the telephone did (4)
    Letters:

− 17. Whooping cough (9)
    Letters:

− 18. Air breathed in and out (11)
    Letters:

− 19. Coal dust in lungs (11)
    Letters:

Final Letter:

Hint: The final letter is the first letter of the topic for this chapter.

Digestive System

KEY TERMS

Absorption
Chylomicrons
Chyme
Mesentery
Peristalsis
Plicae circulares
Rugae

BUILDING VOCABULARY

-algia
amyl-
-ary
-ase
bili-
cec-
cheil-
chole-
col-
cyst-
dent-
-emesis
enter-
gastr-
gingiv-
gloss-
hepat-
lingu-
-orexia
prandi-
proct-
-rrhea
sial-
-stalsis
verm-

CLINICAL TERMS

Anorexia
Aphagia
Ascites
Borborygmus
Bulimia
Cholecystitis
Cholelithiasis
Cirrhosis
Colostomy
Diarrhea
Diverticula
Dysphagia
Edentulous
Emesis
Eructation
Flatus
Gavage
Hematemesis
Intussusception
Laparoscopy
Pyrosis
Volvulus

CLINICAL ABBREVIATIONS

BaE
CLD
CUC
DGE
FOBT
GB
GERD
GI
IBD

CLINICAL ABBREVIATIONS *(cont'd)*

IBS	ORT
LES	PP
NVD	UGI

OUTLINE/OBJECTIVES

Introduction

- List the components of the digestive tract and the accessory organs.
  — The digestive tract includes the mouth, pharynx, esophagus, stomach, small intestine, and large intestine.
  — The accessory organs of the digestive system are the salivary glands, liver, gallbladder, and pancreas.

Functions of the Digestive System

- List six functions of the digestive system.
  — The digestive system prepares nutrients for utilization by the cells of the body.
  — Activities of the digestive system include ingestion, mechanical digestion, chemical digestion, mixing and propelling movements, absorption, and elimination of waste products.

General Structure of the Digestive Tract

- Describe the general histology of the four layers, or tunics, in the digestive tract wall.
  — The basic structure of the wall of the digestive tube is the same throughout the entire length, although there are variations in each region.
  — The wall of the digestive tract consists of a mucosa, submucosa, muscular layer, and an outer adventitia (above the diaphragm) or serosa (below the diaphragm).
  — Nerve plexuses are located in the submucosa and in the muscular layer.

Components of the Digestive Tract

- Describe the features and functions of the oral cavity, teeth, pharynx, and esophagus.
  — The lips and cheeks are muscles covered with epithelium and lined with mucous membrane. The palate is the roof of the mouth. The anterior portion is supported by bone; the posterior portion is muscle and connective tissue.
  — The tongue is composed of skeletal muscle. The dorsal surface is covered with papillae, some of which contain taste buds. The tongue manipulates food in the mouth, contains sensory receptors for taste, and is used in speech.
  — The primary teeth are the deciduous teeth that fall out and are replaced by the secondary or permanent teeth. There are 20 teeth in the complete primary set and 32 teeth in the complete secondary set. The incisors have sharp edges for biting; cuspids have points for grasping and tearing; bicuspids and molars have flat surfaces for grinding. Each tooth has a crown, a neck, and a root. Enamel covers the crown.
  — The pharynx is a passageway that transports food to the esophagus. It is divided into the nasopharynx, oropharynx, and laryngopharynx.
  — The esophagus is posterior to the trachea and anterior to the vertebral column. The lower esophageal sphincter, also called the cardiac sphincter, controls the passage of food into the stomach.

- Name and describe the location of the three major types of salivary glands and describe the functions of the saliva they produce.
  — The parotid, submandibular, and sublingual glands secrete saliva, which contains the enzyme amylase.
  — The parotid glands are anterior and inferior to the ear; the submandibular glands are along the medial surface of the mandible; and the sublingual glands are under the tongue.
  — Saliva contains water, mucus, and amylase.
  — Saliva has a cleansing action, moistens food, dissolves substances for taste, and begins digestion of carbohydrates.
- Describe the structure and histological features of the stomach and its role in digestion.
  — The stomach is divided into a fundus, cardiac region, body, and pyloric region and has a greater curvature and a lesser curvature.
  — The mucosal lining has folds called rugae, and there are three layers of smooth muscle in the wall.
  — Mucous cells secrete mucus; parietal cells secrete hydrochloric acid and intrinsic factor; chief cells secrete pepsinogen; and endocrine cells secrete gastrin.
  — The semifluid mixture of food and gastric juice that leaves the stomach is called chyme.
  — The regulation of gastric secretions is divided into cephalic, gastric, and intestinal phases. Thoughts and smells of food start the cephalic phase; the presence of food in the stomach initiates the gastric phase; and the presence of acid chyme in the small intestine starts the intestinal phase.
  — Relaxation of the pyloric sphincter allows chyme to pass from the stomach into the small intestine. The rate at which stomach emptying occurs depends on the nature of the chyme and the receptivity of the small intestine
- Describe the structure and histological features of the small intestine and its role in digestion and absorption.
  — The absorptive surface area of the small intestine is increased by plicae circulares, villi, and microvilli. Each villus contains a blood capillary network and a lymph capillary called a lacteal.
  — The small intestine is divided into the duodenum, jejunum, and ileum. The duodenum has mucous glands in the submucosa; the jejunum has numerous, long villi; and the ileum has a large number of goblet cells.
  — Cells in the small intestine produce peptidase, which acts on proteins; maltase, sucrase, and lactase, which act on disaccharides; and lipase, which acts on neutral fats.
  — The small intestine produces two hormones, secretin and cholecystokinin. Secretin stimulates the pancreas and cholecystokinin stimulates the gallbladder and digestive enzymes from the pancreas.
  — The presence of chyme in the duodenum stimulates intestinal secretions.
- Describe the structure, histological features, and functions of the large intestine.
  — The mucosa of the large intestine does not have villi, but has a large number of goblet cells. The longitudinal muscle layer is limited to three bands called teniae coli. Haustra and epiploic appendages are also characteristic.
  — The large intestine consists of the cecum, colon, rectum, and anal canal. The colon is divided into the ascending colon on the right side, transverse colon across the anterior abdomen, descending colon on the left, and sigmoid colon across the pelvic brim.
  — The functions of the large intestine include the absorption of water and electrolytes and the elimination of feces.

Accessory Organs of Digestion

- Describe the structure and functions of the liver, gallbladder, and pancreas.

— Externally, the liver is divided into right, left, caudate, and quadrate lobes by the falciform ligament, inferior vena cava (IVC), gallbladder, ligamentum venosum, and ligamentum teres. The porta of the liver is where the hepatic artery and hepatic portal vein enter the liver and the hepatic ducts exit.

— The functional units of the liver are lobules with sinusoids that carry blood from the periphery to the central vein of the lobule. Blood is brought to the liver by the hepatic portal vein and the hepatic artery. The blood from both vessels flows through the sinusoids into the central vein. Central veins merge to form the hepatic veins, which drain into the inferior vena cava.

— The liver has numerous functions that include secretion, synthesis of bile salts, synthesis of plasma proteins, storage, detoxification, excretion, carbohydrate metabolism, lipid metabolism, protein metabolism, and filtering blood.

— The main components of the bile produced by the liver are water, bile salts, bile pigments, and cholesterol. Bile salts act as emulsifying agents in the digestion and absorption of fats. The principal bile pigment is bilirubin, which is formed from the breakdown of hemoglobin. Cholesterol and bile pigments are excreted from the body in the bile.

— The gallbladder is attached to the visceral surface of the liver by the cystic duct, which joins the hepatic duct to form the common bile duct. The common bile duct empties into the duodenum. The gallbladder stores and concentrates the bile.

— The pancreas is retroperitoneal along the posterior body wall and extends from the duodenum to the spleen. Most of the pancreas is exocrine and composed of acinar cells, which produce digestive enzymes. The islets of Langerhans are endocrine and produce insulin and glucagon.

— Pancreatic enzymes include amylase, which acts on starch; trypsin, which acts on proteins; peptidase, which acts on peptides; and lipase, which acts on lipids.

— The hormone secretin stimulates the pancreas to secrete a bicarbonate rich fluid; cholecystokinin stimulates the production of pancreatic enzymes.

Chemical Digestion

• Summarize carbohydrate, protein, and lipid digestion by writing equations that show the intermediate and final products and the enzymes that facilitate the digestive process.
   — Carbohydrates are first broken down into disaccharides by amylase. Disaccharides are then broken down into monosaccharides by sucrase, maltase, and lactase. The end products of carbohydrate digestion are the monosaccharides glucose, fructose, and galactose.
   — Pepsin and trypsin break proteins into shorter chains called peptides. Peptidase breaks peptides into amino acids. The end products of protein digestion are amino acids.
   — Fats are first emulsified by bile. Lipase acts on emulsified fats and breaks them down into monoglycerides and free fatty acids. Monoglycerides and free fatty acids are the end products of lipid digestion.

Absorption

• Compare the absorption of simple sugars and amino acids with that of lipid-related molecules.
   — Most nutrient absorption takes place in the jejunum.
   — Water is absorbed by osmosis in all regions.
   — Simple sugars and amino acids are absorbed into the blood capillaries in the villi of the small intestine, then transported to the liver in the hepatic portal vein.
   — Fatty acids, monoglycerides, and fat-soluble vitamins enter the lacteals in the villi of the small intestine and circulate in the lymph until the lymph enters the left subclavian vein.

LEARNING EXERCISES

Introduction

1. Identify the parts of the digestive system by matching the letters from the figure on the right with the terms on the left. Place an asterisk (*) by the accessory organs.

_____   Esophagus

_____   Gallbladder

_____   Large intestine

_____   Liver

_____   Mouth

_____   Pancreas

_____   Pharynx

_____   Salivary gland

_____   Small intestine

_____   Stomach

Functions of the Digestive System

1. Write the terms that are described by the phrases about the functions of the digestive system.

_____   Process of breaking large food particles into smaller ones

_____   Uses water to break down large molecules into smaller ones

_____   Breaks down complex nonabsorbable molecules into simple usable molecules

_____   Swallowing

_____   Movements that propel food through the digestive tract

_____   Process by which simple molecules from chemical digestion pass through the cell membranes into the blood

_____   Removal of indigestible wastes through the anus

General Structure of the Digestive Tract

1. Match the following descriptions with the correct layer of the digestive tract.

A. mucosa   C. submucosa
B. muscular layer   D. serosa

_____   Innermost layer of the digestive tract wall

_____   Contains blood and lymphatic vessels embedded in loose connective tissue

_____   Responsible for most movements of the digestive tract

_____   Consists of simple columnar epithelium in stomach and intestines

_____   Contains inner circular and outer longitudinal layers

_____   Contains Meissner's plexus of autonomic nerve fibers

_____   Contains the myenteric plexus of autonomic nerve fibers

Components of the Digestive Tract

1. Write the terms that match the phrases about the oral cavity.

_____   Primary muscle in the cheek

_____   Separates oral cavity from nasal cavity

_____   Projection at posterior end of soft palate

_____   Masses of lymphoid tissue at back of tongue

_____   Projections on surface of tongue

_____   Teeth with sharp edges for biting

_____   Teeth with points for grasping and tearing

_____   Largest salivary glands

_____   Glands along medial surface of mandible

_____   Enzyme found in saliva

_____   Functions of saliva (4)

_____

_____

_____

2. Identify the parts of a tooth by matching the letters from the diagram with the correct terms.

_____ Alveolar process

_____ Apical foramen

_____ Cementum

_____ Dentin

_____ Enamel

_____ Gingiva

_____ Pulp cavity

_____ Root canal

3. Write the terms that match the phrases about the pharynx and esophagus.

_____ Opening from oral cavity into pharynx

_____ Most superior region of the pharynx

_____ Region that contains pharyngeal tonsils

_____ Region that contains palatine tonsils

_____ Keeps food from entering nasopharynx

_____ Keeps food from entering laryngopharynx

_____ Tube between pharynx and stomach

_____ Opening in diaphragm for esophagus

_____ Sphincter between esophagus and stomach

4. Identify the regions of the stomach by matching the letters from the diagram with the correct terms. Outline the greater curvature in red and the lesser curvature in blue.

_____ Body

_____ Cardiac region

_____ Duodenum

_____ Fundus

_____ Lower esophageal sphincter

_____ Pyloric sphincter

_____ Pylorus

_____ Rugae

5. Write the terms that match the phrases about the stomach and its secretions.

_____ Acid in gastric juice

_____ Hormone secreted by gastric mucosa

_____ Enzyme in gastric juice

_____ Semifluid mixture of food and gastric juice

_____ Function of intrinsic factor

_____ Factors that influence stomach emptying (2)

_____

6. Match the events in the regulation of gastric secretions with the phase in which they occur.

   A. cephalic phase   B. gastric phase   C. intestinal phase

   _____   Triggered by the passage of chyme into the small intestine

   _____   Begins with thoughts of food

   _____   Begins when food reaches stomach

   _____   Inhibits gastric secretions

   _____   Involves distention of the stomach wall

7. Write the terms that match the phrases about the small intestine and its secretions.

_____ Region adjacent to stomach

_____ Features that increase surface area (3)

_____

_____

_____ Lymph capillary in a villus

_____ Has mucous glands in submucosa

_____ Region with most goblet cells

_____ Activates a pancreatic enzyme

_____ Stimulates release of bile from gallbladder

_____ Stimulates pancreatic release of bicarbonate

_____ Acts on neutral fats

_____ Stimulates pancreatic digestive enzymes

_____ Most important factor for regulating secretions of the small intestine

8. What are the two main functions of the large intestine?

   (a)

   (b)

9. Match the descriptive phrases with the correct terms.

   A. anus
   B. ascending colon
   C. cecum
   D. descending colon
   E. epiploic appendages
   F. haustra
   G. hepatic flexure
   H. ileocecal junction
   I. rectum
   J. sigmoid colon
   K. splenic flexure
   L. teniae coli
   M. transverse colon

   _____ Where small intestine enters the large intestine

   _____ Three bands of longitudinal muscle in large intestine

   _____ Pieces of fat-filled connective tissue attached to colon

   _____ Blind pouch that extends inferiorly from entrance of ileum

   _____ Portion of large intestine on the right side

   _____ Right colonic flexure

   _____ Left colonic flexure

   _____ Portion of large intestine between the two colonic flexures

   _____ Portion of large intestine on the left side

   _____ S-shaped curve across the pelvic brim

   _____ Portion that follows the curvature of the sacrum

   _____ Terminal opening of the digestive tract

   _____ Series of pouches in the large intestine

Accessory Organs of Digestion

1. Write the terms that match the phrases about the liver.

   _____ Attaches liver to anterior abdominal wall

   _____ Region between ligamentum venosum and IVC

   _____ Region between ligamentum teres and gallbladder

   _____ Functional unit of liver

   _____ Venous channels between hepatocytes

   _____ Vessel that carries oxygen-rich blood to the liver

   _____ Vessel that carries nutrient-rich blood to the liver

   _____ Vessel that carries blood away from the liver

_____ Secretory product of the liver

_____ Principal bile pigment

_____ Function of bile salts

_____ Area of bile storage

_____ Duct that attaches gallbladder to liver

_____ Stimulates release of bile from gallbladder

_____ Duct that enters duodenum

_____ Components of a portal triad (3)

_____

_____

2. Write the terms that match the phrases about the pancreas.

_____ Endocrine portion of the pancreas

_____ Exocrine portion of the pancreas

_____ Carries pancreatic enzymes to duodenum

_____ Pancreatic enzyme that acts on starch

_____ Pancreatic enzyme that acts on proteins

_____ Breaks fats into fatty acids and monoglycerides

_____ Hormones that regulate pancreatic secretions (2)

_____

Chemical Digestion

1. Complete the following table about enzymes and their role in digestion.

Enzyme	Source	Digestive Action
	Salivary glands/pancreas	Complex carbohydrates to disaccharides
		Maltose to glucose
Sucrase		
		Lactose to glucose and galactose
	Stomach	Proteins to polypeptides
Trypsin		Proteins to polypeptides
		Peptides to amino acids
		Fats to fatty acids and monoglycerides

2. What are the three monosaccharides that are the end products of carbohydrate digestion?

3. What are the end products of protein digestion?

4. What are the two primary end products of lipid digestion?

Absorption

1. Write the terms that match the phrases about the absorption of nutrients.

_____   Villus vessel that absorbs amino acids and simple sugars

_____   Villus vessel that absorbs triglycerides

_____   Fatty acids coated with bile salts

_____   Triglycerides combined with proteins

_____   Mixture of lymph and digested fats

2. Write the transport process that is responsible for each of the following movements.

_____   Glucose from lumen of small intestine into villus cells

_____   Fructose from lumen of small intestine into villus cells

_____   Water throughout the length of the digestive tract

_____   Most nutrients from villus cells to capillaries and lacteals

REVIEW QUESTIONS

1. Name, in sequence, the regions of the digestive tract.
2. What five activities of the digestive system prepare nutrients for use by the body?
3. Name, in sequence starting with the innermost, the four layers in the wall of the digestive tract.
4. What are the submucosal and myenteric plexuses?
5. Where are the hard and soft palates located? What is the difference in structure between them?
6. What type of muscle makes up the substance of the tongue?
7. What is another name for primary teeth? How many teeth are in this set?
8. What four types of teeth, based on shape, are found in the secondary teeth?
9. What substance covers the crown of a tooth?
10. Where is the largest salivary gland located?
11. What enzyme is found in saliva?
12. What is the fauces?
13. Where is the lower esophageal sphincter located? What is another name for this structure?

14. What are the four regions of the stomach?

15. How does the muscular layer of the stomach differ from that in other regions of the digestive tract?

16. Name the type of cell that produces (a) pepsinogen; (b) hydrochloric acid; (c) gastrin; (d) intrinsic factor.

17. What hormone and what cranial nerve are involved in regulating gastric juice secretion?

18. What sphincter relaxes to allow chyme to pass from the stomach into the small intestine?

19. What three features of the small intestine increase its absorptive surface area?

20. Chyme first enters what part of the small intestine? Secretions from what two glands also enter this region?

21. Which region of the small intestine has (a) the longest villi; (b) an opening for the cystic duct; (c) the most goblet cells; (d) an opening for the pancreatic duct; (e) mucous glands in the submucosa?

22. What is the function of (a) maltase; (b) peptidase; (c) secretin; (d) enterokinase; (e) cholecystokinin?

23. What is the most important factor that regulates the secretion of enzymes and hormones in the small intestine?

24. What are teniae coli, haustra, and epiploic appendages?

25. Between which two parts of the large intestine is the hepatic flexure located? Splenic flexure?

26. Which anal sphincter is controlled voluntarily?

27. What are two functions of the large intestine?

28. What ligament attaches the anterior surface of the liver to the anterior abdominal wall?

29. Name three boundaries of the caudate lobe of the liver.

30. What are the components of a portal triad?

31. What two blood vessels bring blood to the liver sinusoids?

32. What function of the liver is specifically related to digestion?

33. What two substances are excreted in the bile?

34. What hormone stimulates the gallbladder to contract?

35. Where is the pancreas located?

36. What cells in the pancreas secrete enzymes that are important in digestion?

37. What is the function of (a) amylase; (b) trypsin; (c) peptidase; (d) lipase?

38. Use the terms secretin and cholecystokinin in a description of the regulation of pancreatic secretion.

39. What are the end products of carbohydrate digestion?

40. Name two enzymes that are involved in the digestion of proteins into peptides.

41. What are the end products of lipid digestion?

42. What structures absorb simple sugars and amino acids in the small intestine? What structures absorb fatty acids and monoglycerides?

CHAPTER QUIZ

1. Which of the following terms refers to chemical digestion? (a) mastication; (b) hydrolysis; (c) peristalsis; (d) defecation; (e) deglutition.

2. Starting from the inside, or lumen, the sequence of layers in the wall of the gastrointestinal tract is (a) serosa, mucosa, submucosa, muscular; (b) mucosa, submucosa, inner longitudinal muscle, outer circular muscle; (c) serosa, muscular, submucosa, mucosa; (d) mucosa, submucosa, muscular, serosa; (e) inner muscle, submucosa, mucosa, outer muscular.

3. How many more teeth are there in a complete permanent set than in a complete deciduous set?

4. True or False: The largest of the salivary glands is the parotid gland, which is located in the oropharynx.

5. Match each of the following descriptions with the appropriate structure. Each description has only one response. Responses are to be used only once and not all responses will be used.

   A. duodenum
   B. fauces
   C. fundus
   D. haustra
   E. hepatic flexure
   F. ileocecal sphincter
   G. ileum
   H. jejunum

   I. lower esophageal sphincter
   J. plicae circulares
   K. pyloric sphincter
   L. pylorus
   M. rugae
   N. splenic flexure
   O. teniae coli

   _____ Opening from the oral cavity into the pharynx

   _____ Portion of the stomach that is superior to the entrance of the esophagus

   _____ Circular band of muscle at the exit from the stomach

   _____ Circular folds of mucosa in the small intestine

   _____ Circular band of muscle between the esophagus and stomach

   _____ Curve between the ascending colon and the transverse colon

   _____ Longitudinal folds of mucosa in the stomach

   _____ Longitudinal muscle bands in the large intestine

   _____ Shortest part of the small intestine

   _____ Circular band of muscle between the small intestine and large intestine

6. Match the following actions with the appropriate enzyme or hormone. Some responses may be used more than once and others may not be used at all.

   A. amylase   D. secretin
   B. cholecystokinin   E. trypsin
   C. maltase

   _____ Breaks carbohydrates into disaccharides

   _____ Stimulates secretion of bile

   _____ Acts on a disaccharide

   _____ Stimulates secretion of bicarbonate from pancreas

   _____ Breaks proteins into peptides

   _____ Stimulates secretion of enzymes from the pancreas

7. Which of the following represents the correct sequence of blood flow from the gastrointestinal tract through the liver? (a) hepatic artery, sinusoids, hepatic portal vein, hepatic vein, inferior vena cava; (b) hepatic portal vein, sinusoids, central vein, hepatic vein, inferior vena cava; (c) hepatic vein, sinusoids, central vein, hepatic portal vein, inferior vena cava; (d) hepatic portal vein, hepatic vein, sinusoids, central vein, inferior vena cava; (e) hepatic vein, hepatic portal vein, central vein, sinusoids, inferior vena cava

8. What function of the liver pertains to the digestion of fats?

9. What two secretory ducts empty into the duodenum?

10. The following six items are end products of digestion. Indicate whether each is a product of carbohydrate (C), protein (P), or fat (F) digestion and whether it is absorbed by the blood capillaries (B) or lacteals (L) of the villi. Each end product should be designated by a C, P, or an F, and by a B or an L.

    C, P, F   B or L

    _____ _____ Glucose

    _____ _____ Amino acids

    _____ _____ Monoglycerides

    _____ _____ Fructose

    _____ _____ Fatty acids

    _____ _____ Galactose

USING CLINICAL KNOWLEDGE

1. Match the definitions on the left with the correct term from the column on the right by placing the corresponding letter in the space before the definition. Not all terms will be used.

_____	Folds in the stomach mucosa	A. Anorexia
_____	Semifluid mixture of food and gastric juice that enters the small intestine	B. Antidiarrheals
		C. Ascites
_____	Twisting of the bowel that causes an obstruction	D. Bulimia
_____	An emotional disorder characterized by binge eating	E. Chyle
		F. Chyme
_____	Increase rate of fecal movement through colon	G. Hematemesis
_____	Folds in the mucosa and submucosa of small intestine	H. Laxatives
		I. Plicae circulares
_____	Blood in the vomit	J. Pyrosis
_____	Heartburn; regurgitation of stomach acid into the esophagus	K. Rugae
		L. Volvulus
_____	Drugs that reduce peristalsis in the intestines	
_____	Accumulation of serous fluid in the peritoneal cavity	

2. Write the meaning of the following abbreviations.

_____ GERD

_____ NVD

_____ GI

_____ GB

_____ FOBT

3. Spelling is important in scientific and medical applications because only one or two incorrect letters may change the meaning. Circle the correctly spelled word for each of the following pairs.

esophageal	esophogeal
postpandial	postprandial
glosopharyngeal	glossopharyngeal
masetter	masseter
monoglycerides	monoglyserides

4. Write the meaning of the underlined portion of each word on the line preceding the word.

_____ chole cystectomy

_____ enteropathy

_____ cholecystectomy

_____ gingivitis

_____ hepatomegaly

_____ anorexia

_____ sialadenectomy

_____ sialadenectomy

_____ sialadenectomy

_____ hematemesis

5. Dee Jeston had a salivary gland removed by surgery. Select the medical term for this procedure from the list in question #4.

6. Janie Student's baby was vomiting almost continuously. Use your knowledge of word parts to write the medical term for this condition of excessive vomiting.

7. Drew Deenum complained of pain in and around the rectum and anus. Use your knowledge of word parts to write the medical term for this condition

FUN AND GAMES

This is a variation of the word game Hangman. Guess any letter for the first word and find the number that corresponds to that letter in the Letter Chart at the bottom of the page. Then find that same number above the line that divides each cell in the Position Chart on the right. If the letter you guessed appears in the word, its position is given by the number or numbers below the line that divides each cell in the Position Chart. If the letter does not appear in the word, 0 will be indicated under the line. If the letter you guessed does not appear in the word, start drawing a stick person on a gallows – first a head, then a body, followed by two arms and two legs. You are allotted six wrong guesses before you are hanged. Clue: Words are from this chapter on the digestive system.

Words

#1 — — — — — — —
  1 2 3 4 5 6 7

#2 — — — — — — — —
  1 2 3 4 5 6 7 8

#3 — — — — — — — —
  1 2 3 4 5 6 7 8

#4 — — — — — — — —
  1 2 3 4 5 6 7 8

#5 — — — — — — — — —
  1 2 3 4 5 6 7 8 9

#6 — — — — — — — — — —
  1 2 3 4 5 6 7 8 9 10

#7 — — — — — — — — — — —
  1 2 3 4 5 6 7 8 9 10 11

#8 — — — — — — — — — — —
  1 2 3 4 5 6 7 8 9 10 11

#9 — — — — — — — — — — —
  1 2 3 4 5 6 7 8 9 10 11

#10 — — — — — — — — — — —
  1 2 3 4 5 6 7 8 9 10 11

Letters Missed

| _ | _ | _ | _ | _ | _ |

| _ | _ | _ | _ | _ | _ |

| _ | _ | _ | _ | _ | _ |

| _ | _ | _ | _ | _ | _ |

| _ | _ | _ | _ | _ | _ |

| _ | _ | _ | _ | _ | _ |

| _ | _ | _ | _ | _ | _ |

| _ | _ | _ | _ | _ | _ |

| _ | _ | _ | _ | _ | _ |

| _ | _ | _ | _ | _ | _ |

Position Chart

1	2	3	4	5
4	0	9	5, 7	0
6	**7**	**8**	**9**	**10**
0	1, 3	0	0	5
11	**12**	**13**	**14**	**15**
3, 6	0	4, 8	2, 9	0
16	**17**	**18**	**19**	**20**
6	0	6, 9	4	5,9,11
21	**22**	**23**	**24**	**25**
0	2, 5	0	0	5
26	**27**	**28**	**29**	**30**
6, 10	0	8	0	3
31	**32**	**33**	**34**	**35**
0	4, 10	0	0	0
36	**37**	**38**	**39**	**40**
0	0	5, 7	0	7, 9
41	**42**	**43**	**44**	**45**
0	1	0	5, 9	0
46	**47**	**48**	**49**	**50**
11	0	3, 6	0	0
51	**52**	**53**	**54**	**55**
2	0	0	0	2, 7
56	**57**	**58**	**59**	**60**
0	1	0	2	0
61	**62**	**63**	**64**	**65**
8	0	6, 8	0	0
66	**67**	**68**	**69**	**70**
0	1, 4	0	0	8
71	**72**	**73**	**74**	**75**
10	0	0	0	7
76	**77**	**78**	**79**	**80**
0	0	3	0	0
81	**82**	**83**	**84**	**85**
3	0	0	0	0

Letter Chart

	A	B	C	D	E	F	G	H	I	J	K	L	M	N	O	P	Q	R	S	T	U	V	W	X	Y	Z
#1	75	2	50	85	5	23	67	2	22	56	5	72	39	81	47	17	8	83	49	31	58	16	6	77	82	34
#2	68	33	72	8	24	2	83	36	53	41	84	11	50	37	59	69	50	41	61	5	38	67	24	64	5	53
#3	47	9	66	21	81	42	60	35	76	8	35	16	61	19	5	49	62	51	79	69	4	45	8	12	31	85
#4	23	58	76	67	10	82	66	49	12	2	79	23	70	16	30	6	41	34	84	27	55	27	64	9	17	45
#5	18	12	27	57	34	10	75	25	28	85	39	33	12	72	56	1	65	56	78	5	74	69	50	23	51	21
#6	65	53	33	76	14	79	61	52	10	73	29	52	74	26	75	7	8	62	1	43	80	36	82	43	80	39
#7	23	82	9	42	51	45	81	15	40	58	77	19	68	46	71	82	52	39	27	63	25	17	60	21	2	54
#8	75	34	24	84	59	35	15	66	32	64	84	61	9	27	80	42	29	78	20	16	73	31	77	37	85	74
#9	55	43	16	77	37	43	68	85	44	77	24	45	57	46	71	15	37	6	78	13	54	36	43	17	65	60
#10	21	67	29	47	36	83	70	52	35	56	15	54	3	41	22	73	31	48	46	33	71	6	83	29	75	62

17

Metabolism and Nutrition

KEY TERMS

Acetyl-CoA
Anabolism
Basal metabolic rate
Beta oxidation
Catabolism
Citric acid cycle
Complete protein
Core temperature
Deamination
Gluconeogenesis
Glycogenesis
Glycogenolysis
Glycolysis
Lipogenesis
Thermogenesis

BUILDING VOCABULARY

ana-
-bol-
cata-
-clysis
fruct-
-gen-
lys-
mal-
neo-
nutri-
-pepsia
prote-
pyr-
therm-
-tion
vita-

CLINICAL TERMS

Achlorhydria
Alimentation
Celiac disease
Heat exhaustion
Hypervitaminosis
Hypothermia
Jaundice
Kwashiorkor
Malabsorption syndrome
Malnutrition
Marasmus
Pica
Undernutrition

CLINICAL ABBREVIATIONS

AMS
ASAP
BBT
BED
BMI
BMR
DAT
D/W
FFA
FUO
HDL
LDL
MNT
temp
TNP
TPR

OUTLINE/OBJECTIVES

Metabolism of Absorbed Nutrients

- Define the terms metabolism and nutrition.
  - — Metabolism is the sum of all the chemical reactions in the body. Within a cell, the reactions are called cellular metabolism. Enzymes speed up the reactions.
  - — Nutrition is the acquisition, assimilation, and utilization of the nutrients that are contained in food. The utilization of the nutrients is a part of metabolism.
- Distinguish between anabolism and catabolism.
  - — Anabolism uses energy to build large molecules from smaller ones. Dehydration synthesis is a type of anabolic reaction in which a water molecule is removed when a larger molecule is synthesized from two smaller ones.
  - — Catabolism releases energy when large molecules break down into smaller ones. Catabolic reactions within the cell that release energy for use by the cell are termed cellular respiration.
- Describe the basic steps in glycolysis, the citric acid cycle, and electron transport.
  - — Cellular respiration utilizes the absorbed end products of digestion and stores the energy in the high energy bonds of adenosine triphosphate (ATP).
  - — The first step in the catabolism of glucose is glycolysis, which takes place in the cytoplasm and is anaerobic. Two pyruvic acid molecules are produced from one glucose molecule and there is a net gain of 2 ATP.
  - — If oxygen is present, pyruvic acid enters the mitochondria for the aerobic phase of cellular respiration. The pyruvic acid is incorporated into acetyl CoA, which enters the citric acid cycle. Hydrogen ions produced in the citric acid cycle combine with oxygen in the electron transport chain to produce water and ATP. The complete breakdown of glucose produces 36 – 38 ATP.
- Define glycogen, glycogenesis, glycogenolysis, and gluconeogenesis.
  - — Glycogen is the storage form of glucose. Glycogen is synthesized from glucose by glycogenesis. Glycogenolysis is the breakdown of glycogen into glucose and gluconeogenesis is the production of glucose from noncarbohydrate sources.
- Describe the pathway by which proteins are utilized in the body.
  - — The end products of protein digestion are amino acids. Amino acids are used to synthesize proteins to build new tissues and replace damaged tissues. They are also used to synthesize hemoglobin, hormones, enzymes, and plasma proteins.
  - — Amino acids may be used as an energy source by removing the amino group (deamination). The resulting keto acid enters the citric acid cycle to produce energy.
- Describe the pathway by which fatty acids are broken down to produce ATP.
  - — The end products of lipid digestion are monoglycerides and fatty acids, which are an important source of energy.
  - — Fatty acids are catabolized by beta oxidation, which removes 2-carbon segments from fatty acid chains and converts the segments to acetyl CoA. The acetyl CoA enters the citric acid cycle to produce ATP.
- Name two key molecules in the metabolism and interconversion of carbohydrates, proteins, and fats.
  - — The end products of carbohydrate, protein, and lipid metabolism can be interconverted when necessary. Pyruvic acid and acetyl CoA are key molecules in the metabolism and interconversion of carbohydrates, proteins, and fats.
- Explain how energy from food is measured.
  - — Energy from food is measured in calories. One calorie is the amount of energy required to raise the temperature of one kilogram of water from 14° Celsius to 15° Celsius.
- Define basal metabolism and state four factors that influence it.

— Basal metabolism is the energy that is necessary to keep the body functioning at a minimal level. It is influenced by sex, muscle mass, age, hormones, and body temperature. It is a balance between energy expenditure and energy production.
— Increasing physical activity increases energy expenditure in the body. Physical activity is the only means of voluntarily controlling energy expenditure.
— Thermogenesis is the production of heat through the assimilation of food.
— Digestion, absorption, and metabolism use chemical energy, and heat energy is produced.

Basic Elements of Nutrition

- List the functions of carbohydrates, proteins, and fats in the body.
    — Carbohydrates provide energy, add bulk to the diet, and are used to synthesize other compounds.
    — Proteins provide structure, regulate body processes, and provide energy.
    — Lipids are an important source of energy, provide essential fatty acids, transport vitamins, are components of certain structural elements, provide heat insulation, and form protective cushions.
- State the caloric value of carbohydrates, proteins, and fats.
    — One gram of pure carbohydrate yields 4 calories of energy.
    — One gram of protein yields 4 calories of energy.
    — One gram of fat yields 9 calories of energy.
- Explain the importance of fiber in the diet.
    — Fiber adds bulk to the diet, enhances absorption of nutrients, and helps move the feces in the large intestine. Many diseases are related to decreased dietary fiber.
- Distinguish between essential and nonessential amino acids and between complete and incomplete proteins.
    — Essential amino acids must be supplied in the diet; they cannot be synthesized in the body. Nonessential amino acids can be synthesized from other amino acids that are available.
    — Complete proteins contain all the essential amino acids. Incomplete proteins lack one or more of the essential amino acids. Incomplete proteins should be eaten in combinations that provide all the essential amino acids.
- Discuss the functions of vitamins, minerals, and water in the body.
    — Vitamins are organic molecules that are necessary for good health. Many vitamins are part of enzyme molecules, which are incomplete without the vitamin portion. These enzymes are necessary for the chemical reactions throughout the body.
    — Minerals are inorganic substances that are necessary in small amounts to maintain good health. They are obtained from plants since the plants absorb them from the soil. Some minerals are components of body structures; some are parts of enzyme molecules; others help control fluid levels; and others become part of larger organic molecules.
    — Water is an essential component of the diet. The average adult requires about 2.5 liters of water every day. Water is an integral part of body cells, provides a medium for chemical reactions, is a transport medium, is a lubricant, and helps maintain body temperature.

Body Temperature

- Distinguish between core temperature and shell temperature.
    — Core temperature is the temperature of the internal organs; shell temperature is the temperature at the body surface.
- Explain three ways in which core temperature is maintained when the environmental temperature is cold.

— Heat is produced by the catabolism of nutrients. The body produces additional heat by muscular contraction (shivering) and increasing metabolic rate (hormones). Heat is conserved by constriction of cutaneous blood vessels, which keeps the blood warmer by keeping it away from the cold surface of the body.

* State four ways in which heat is lost from the body.
  — Heat is lost from the body through radiation, conduction, convection, and evaporation.
* Describe the general mechanism by which the body maintains core temperature and identify the region of the brain that integrates this mechanism.
  — Body temperature is regulated by a homeostatic negative feedback mechanism that is integrated by the hypothalamus of the brain.

LEARNING EXERCISES

Metabolism of Absorbed Nutrients

1. Write the terms that match the given definitions.

   _____ Total of all chemical reactions in the body

   _____ Chemical reactions within cells to produce energy

   _____ Substances that speed up physiologic reactions

   _____ Acquisition and utilization of nutrients

2. Match the following terms with the correct definitions or descriptive phrases.

A. acetyl CoA	F. deamination	K. glycogenolysis
B. aerobic	G. gluconeogenesis	L. glycolysis
C. anaerobic	H. glucose	M. lactic acid
D. beta oxidation	I. glycogen	N. lipogenesis
E. cytoplasm	J. glycogenesis	O. mitochondria

   _____ Most important simple sugar in cellular metabolism

   _____ Term that means oxygen is not required

   _____ Reactions in which glucose is split into two molecules of pyruvic acid

   _____ Fate of pyruvic acid in absence of oxygen

   _____ Term that means oxygen is required

   _____ Molecule that enters the citric acid cycle

   _____ Storage form of glucose

   _____ Location of glycolysis reactions

   _____ Location of citric acid cycle reactions

   _____ Conversion of glucose to glycogen

   _____ Conversion of glucose to fat

   _____ Conversion of glycogen into glucose

   _____ Conversion of noncarbohydrates to glucose

   _____ Principal reaction that prepares amino acids for use as an energy source

   _____ Reactions that convert fatty acids to acetyl CoA

3. State six uses of the proteins that are synthesized in the body. Do not include their possible use as an energy source.

   (a)

   (b)

   (c)

   (d)

   (e)

   (f)

4. What are the two key molecules in the interconversion of carbohydrates, proteins, and fats?

5. Define or explain what is meant by the nutritional calorie or kilocalorie.

6. List the three uses of energy in the body. Draw a circle around the one that accounts for most of the energy used. Place an asterisk (*) by the one that can be controlled voluntarily.

   (a)

   (b)

   (c)

Basic Elements of Nutrition

1. Indicate whether each of the following most closely applies to carbohydrates, lipids, or proteins. Use C = carbohydrates, L = lipids, and P = proteins.

   _____ Primary energy source   _____ Glucose

   _____ Regulate body processes   _____ Concentrated energy

   _____ Major component of cell membranes   _____ Fiber

   _____ Transport vitamins A, D, E, K   _____ Hormones, enzymes

   _____ Add bulk to the diet   _____ Steroids

   _____ Fatty acids   _____ Glycogen

   _____ Provide insulation and protection   _____ Triglycerides

   _____ Provide structure   _____ Amino acids

2. How many calories are in each of the following?

_____ 1 gram pure carbohydrate   _____ 5 grams carbohydrate

_____ 1 gram pure protein   _____ 4 grams protein

_____ 1 gram pure fat   _____ 3 grams fat

3. Complete the following paragraph by writing the correct words in the blanks.

Amino acids that cannot be synthesized in the body and must be supplied in the diet are called

_____ amino acids. A protein that contains all of these amino acids

is called a _____ protein. Other proteins, called incomplete pro-

teins, should be eaten in combinations to provide all of the _____

amino acids.

4. Complete the following paragraph by writing the correct words in the blanks.

The American Heart Association recommends that no more than _____

of the daily calorie intake should be in the form of fats. Further, it recommends a reduction

in the amount of saturated fats in the diet. In general, foods that are high in saturated fats are

also high in _____. Cholesterol intake should be limited to less than

_____ _____ per day.

5. Classify the following vitamins as being either water soluble or fat soluble. Use W for water soluble and F for fat soluble.

_____ Thiamine   _____ Vitamin A   _____ Vitamin D

_____ Niacin   _____ Vitamin C   _____ Riboflavin

6. Indicate whether each of the following most closely applies to uses of vitamins, minerals, or water in the body. Use V = vitamins, M = minerals, and W = water.

_____ Medium for chemical reactions   _____ Incorporated into bones and teeth

_____ Release energy from nutrients   _____ Maintenance of body temperature

_____ Nucleic acid synthesis   _____ Regulation of body fluid levels

Body Temperature

1. Match the following terms with the correct definitions or descriptive phrases about body temperature.

A. blood
B. constriction of vessels in skin
C. core temperature
D. epinephrine
E. heat

F. hypothalamus
G. perspiration
H. radiation
I. shell temperature
J. shivering

_____   By-product of cellular metabolism

_____   Location of the body's thermostat

_____   Temperature of internal organs

_____   Heat-producing hormone

_____   Distributes heat through the body

_____   Methods of increasing body heat (2)

_____

_____   Methods of releasing body heat (2)

_____

_____   Temperature at the body surface

REVIEW QUESTIONS

1. What is the relationship between metabolism and nutrition?

2. What group of reactions releases chemical energy in the cell and what molecule represents this chemical energy?

3. Where in the cell does glycolysis take place and what are the end products?

4. What happens to pyruvic acid in the aerobic phase of cellular respiration and where does this occur?

5. How do glycogenesis and glycogenolysis help maintain a constant blood glucose level?

6. What is the primary purpose of amino acids in the body?

7. What type of reaction prepares amino acids so they can be used as a source of energy?

8. What type of chemical reaction is involved in the catabolism of fatty acids? What is the end product of this process?

9. What are the two key molecules in gluconeogenesis?

10. What is the difference between basal metabolic rate and total metabolic rate?

11. Which component of energy expenditure can be controlled voluntarily?

12. Compare the amounts of energy that can be obtained from one gram of carbohydrate, protein, and fat.

13. What is the form in which carbohydrate is carried in the blood?

14. Give a common food source for (a) fructose; (b) sucrose; (c) lactose; (d) maltose.

15. Starch and fiber are derived from plant sources. What is their difference in terms of utilization?

16. In what ways do proteins help regulate body processes?

17. Why are certain amino acids termed essential?

18. What is lacking in an incomplete protein?

19. What category of nutrients represents a concentrated energy source?

20. What is the American Heart Association's recommendation regarding dietary intake of saturated fats? What common food sources are high in saturated fats?

21. What vitamins require fats for absorption and utilization?

22. Why are vitamins and minerals necessary in the diet?

23. What are the primary food sources of minerals?

24. Why is water essential to good health?

25. What are homeotherms?

26. Which is greater—core temperature or shell temperature?

27. What is the main source of heat to maintain core temperature?

28. What accounts for most of the heat loss from the body?

29. Where is the body's thermostat located?

CHAPTER QUIZ

1. For each of the following, indicate whether it refers to anabolism or to catabolism. Use A = anabolism and C = catabolism.

   _____ Releases energy

   _____ Cellular respiration

   _____ Dehydration synthesis

   _____ Breaks large molecules into smaller ones

2. Which one of the following is *not* a characteristic of glycolysis? (a) anaerobic; (b) occurs in mitochondria; (c) produces ATP; (d) glucose is converted to pyruvic acid

3. Which one of the following is *not* a characteristic of the aerobic phase of cellular respiration? (a) occurs in mitochondria; (b) called the citric acid cycle; (c) end product is acetyl CoA; (d) releases energy in the form of ATP and heat

4. What large carbohydrate molecule represents the storage form of glucose in humans?

5. For each of the following, indicate whether it is a feature or characteristic of deamination or beta oxidation. Use D = deamination and B = beta oxidation.

   _____ A reaction in protein catabolism

   _____ Breaks off two-carbon segments from fatty acid chains

   _____ Produces ammonia

   _____ A reaction in the utilization of amino acids for energy

   _____ Produces acetyl CoA

   _____ A step in the conversion of amino acids to glucose

   _____ A reaction in lipid catabolism

6. Which is greater: energy used for basal metabolism or energy used for thermogenesis?

7. How many calories are derived from 8 grams of carbohydrate? How many grams of fat give the same number of calories?

8. Match each description with the appropriate carbohydrate.

   _____ A monosaccharide   A. fiber

   _____ Nondigestible complex polysaccharide   B. glucose

   _____ Formed from two glucose molecules   C. maltose

   _____ Glucose storage form in plants   D. starch

   _____ Table sugar   E. sucrose

9. Name the vitamin that is important for

   _____ Collagen synthesis

   _____ Formation of pigments in the retina

   _____ Synthesis of clotting factors

   _____ Formation of erythrocytes

   _____ Synthesis of DNA

10. In response to a cold environment, (a) the cutaneous blood vessels dilate so you feel warmer; (b) the metabolic rate deceases to conserve heat; (c) core temperature decreases before the shell temperature decreases; (d) epinephrine and norepinephrine promote heat production

USING CLINICAL KNOWLEDGE

1. Match the definitions on the left with the correct term from the column on the right by placing the corresponding letter in the space before the definition. Not all terms will be used.

_____	Production of heat in response to food intake	A. Achlorhydria
_____	Amount of energy necessary to maintain life at a minimal level	B. Basal metabolic rate
_____	Intravenous approach to nutrition	C. Core temperature
_____	Yellow skin color caused by excessive bilirubin	D. Enteral nutrition
_____	A state of poor nourishment	E. Jaundice
_____	Temperature of internal organs	F. Kwashiorkor
_____	Nutrients enter some region of the GI tract	G. Malnutrition
_____	Deficiency of protein and calorie intake	H. Marasmus
_____	Absence of HCl in gastric secretions	I. Parenteral nutrition
_____	Inadequate food intake	J. Shell temperature
		K. Thermogenesis
		L. Undernutrition

2. Write the meaning of the following abbreviations.

_____ BED

_____ BMR

_____ HDL

_____ TPN

_____ BMI

3. Spelling is important in scientific and medical applications because only one or two incorrect letters may change the meaning. Circle the correctly spelled word for each of the following pairs.

anairobic	anaerobic
asetyl-CoA	acetyl-CoA
triglycerides	triglyserides
homeotherm	homotherm
glucogenolysis	glycogenolysis

4. Write the meaning of the underlined portion of each word on the line preceding the word.

_____ <u>clyst</u>er

_____ <u>fruct</u>ose

_____ dys<u>pep</u>sia

_____ <u>ana</u>bolism

_____ glyco<u>lys</u>is

_____ <u>cata</u>bolism

_____ <u>mal</u>nutrition

_____ <u>pyr</u>ogenic

_____ <u>vita</u>min

_____ gluco<u>neo</u>genesis

5. Wally O. Beese went to his PCP for a follow-up after having some blood work done. The PCP explained that he was at risk for CAD because his blood showed elevated levels of "bad" cholesterol. He also suggested that Wally try to lose weight by increasing his metabolic rate and by reducing his intake of fatty foods such as French fries, butter, and potato chips.

a. What is CAD?

b. What is the medical term for "bad" cholesterol?

c. Why does "bad" cholesterol increase the risk of CAD?

d. What part of the total metabolic rate can be voluntarily controlled?

e. Why do fats cause more weight gain than an equal quantity of CHO?

FUN AND GAMES

The object of this puzzle is to accumulate as many points as possible for the words you select as answers for the clues. To do the puzzle, answer each clue with a single word and write that word in the space by the clue. Each letter of the alphabet is assigned point values as indicated. Using these point values, add up your score for each answer. Each clue has more than one possible answer and you should try to choose the one that gives the highest point value. Finally, add the ten individual scores to get your total score for the puzzle. For fair play, use single word answers only and avoid answers, such as lactic acid and beta oxidation, that contain two words. Try competing with your classmates to see who can get the highest score! Have fun!

A = 1	B = 2	C = 2	D = 2	E = 1	F = 3	G = 3
H = 3	I = 1	J = 5	K = 4	L = 2	M = 2	N = 1
O = 1	P = 3	Q = 5	R = 1	S = 1	T = 1	U = 1
V = 4	W = 4	X = 5	Y = 3	Z = 5		

Clue	Single Word Answer	Points
1. A phase of metabolism	_____	_____
2. A process that breaks down or produces glucose	_____	_____
3. A hexose monosaccharide	_____	_____
4. A disaccharide	_____	_____
5. A complex polysaccharide	_____	_____
6. A lipid	_____	_____
7. Mechanism of heat loss	_____	_____
8. Mineral required in the diet	_____	_____
9. One of the B vitamins	_____	_____
10. Protein catabolism reaction	_____	_____

18

Urinary System and Body Fluids

KEY TERMS

Acidosis
Alkalosis
Extracellular fluid
Glomerular capsule
Interstitial fluid
Intracellular fluid
Intravascular fluid
Juxtaglomerular apparatus
Nephron
Renal tubule

BUILDING VOCABULARY

-atresia
azot-
caly-
-cele
-chrom-
-continence
cyst-
-ectasy
-etic
juxta-
ket-
lith-
mict-
neph-
noct-
olig-
peri-
-pexy
-phraxis
pyel-
ren-
-rrhaphy
-ur-

CLINICAL TERMS

Anuria
Azotemia
Blood urea nitrogen
Catheterization
Cystoscopy
Dialysis
Diuresis
Diuretic
Dysuria
Enuresis
Intravenous pyelogram
Lithotripsy
Nephrectomy
Nephritis
Nocturia
Oliguria
Polyuria

CLINICAL ABBREVIATIONS

ARF
BUN
cath
CBI
creat
CRF
CUG
ERPF
ESRD
GFR
IVP
KUB
PKU
RPF
TUR
UA
UTI

OUTLINE/OBJECTIVES

Components of the Urinary System

- State six functions of the urinary system.
  - The urinary system rids the body of waste materials, regulates fluid volume, maintains electrolyte concentrations in body fluids, controls blood pH, secretes erythropoietin, and secretes renin.
- Describe the location and structural features of the kidneys.
  - The components of the urinary system are the kidneys, ureters, urinary bladder, and urethra.
  - The kidneys are retroperitoneal against the posterior abdominal wall, between the levels of the twelfth thoracic and third lumbar vertebrae.
  - An indentation called the hilus leads to the renal sinus. The renal artery, renal vein, and ureter penetrate the kidney at the hilus.
  - The kidney is enclosed by a capsule and surrounded by perirenal fat.
  - Internally, the renal cortex, renal medulla, pyramids, renal columns, papillae, calyces, and pelvis are visible.
- Draw and label a diagrammatic representation of a nephron.
  - The nephron is the functional unit of the kidney and consists of a renal corpuscle and a renal tubule.
  - The renal corpuscle consists of a glomerulus and a glomerular capsule.
  - The renal tubule consists of a proximal convoluted tubule, the nephron loop with descending and ascending limbs, and a distal convoluted tubule.
  - The nephron loop is the only part of a nephron located in the pyramids. The other portions are in the cortex.
  - Urine passes from the nephrons into collecting ducts, then into the minor calyces.
  - Collecting ducts are located in the pyramids.
- Name the two parts of the juxtaglomerular apparatus and state where they are located.
  - The juxtaglomerular apparatus consists of modified cells where the ascending limb of the nephron loop (macula densa) comes in contact with the afferent arteriole (juxtaglomerular cells).
  - The juxtaglomerular cells secrete renin
- Trace the pathway of blood flow through the kidney from the renal artery to the renal vein.
  - Blood flows through the kidney in the sequence: renal artery, segmental arteries, interlobar arteries, arcuate arteries, interlobular arteries, afferent arteriole, glomerulus, efferent arteriole, peritubular capillaries.
  - From the capillaries back to the renal vein, the sequence is peritubular capillaries, interlobular veins, arcuate veins, interlobar veins, segmental veins, and renal vein.
- Describe the location, structure, and function of the ureter, urinary bladder, and urethra.
  - The ureter transports urine from the kidney to the urinary bladder and is continuous with the renal pelvis.
  - As it leaves the kidney, the ureter descends along the posterior abdominal wall and is retroperitoneal.
  - The ureters enter the urinary bladder on the posterior and inferior surface.
  - The urinary bladder is posterior to the symphysis pubis and below the parietal peritoneum in the pelvic cavity.
  - The lining of the urinary bladder is a mucous membrane with folds called rugae. The smooth muscle in the wall is the detrusor muscle.
  - The trigone, in the floor of the urinary bladder, is outlined by the two ureters and the internal urethral orifice.
  - Micturition is the act of expelling urine from the bladder.
  - The urethra transports urine from the bladder to the exterior of the body.

— The flow is controlled by two sphincters. The internal sphincter is located where the urethra leaves the bladder and is smooth muscle. The external sphincter is located where the urethra penetrates the pelvic floor and is skeletal muscle.

— In females the urethra is short. In males it is longer and extends the length of the penis. The male urethra is divided into the prostatic urethra, membranous urethra, and the spongy urethra.

— The urethra opens to the exterior through the external urethral orifice.

Urine Formation

• Describe each of the three basic steps in urine formation.
  — The work of the kidneys is accomplished through the formation of urine, which involves glomerular filtration, tubular reabsorption, and tubular secretion.
  — In glomerular filtration, plasma components cross the filtration membrane from the glomerulus into the glomerular capsule.
  — Tubular reabsorption moves substances from the filtrate into the blood in the capillaries and reduces the volume of urine. Most of the solutes are reabsorbed by active transport mechanisms. Water is reabsorbed by osmosis in all parts of the tubule except the ascending limb of the nephron loop, which is impermeable to water.
  — Tubular secretion adds substances to the urine. Hydrogen ions, potassium ions, creatinine, histamine, and penicillin are examples of substances that are added to the urine by tubular secretion.
• Identify three different types of pressure that affect the rate of glomerular filtration and describe how these interact.
  — The rate of glomerular filtration depends on the net filtration pressure. This pressure is the result of the interaction of the blood pressure in the glomerulus, hydrostatic pressure in the capsule, and osmotic pressure in the blood.
• Explain why some substances, such as glucose, have limited reabsorption and what happens when concentration exceeds this limit.
  — Reabsorption of some solutes is limited by carrier molecules. When the concentration of these solutes exceeds renal threshold, the excess appears in the urine.
• Explain how kidney function has a role in maintaining blood concentration, blood volume, and blood pressure.
  — By altering the concentration and volume of urine, the kidneys have a major role in maintaining blood concentration, volume, and pressure.
• Name two hormones that affect kidney function and explain the effect of each one.
  — Aldosterone increases sodium reabsorption in the kidney tubules. This causes sodium retention, and secondarily, water retention. This will also increase blood volume and blood pressure.
  — Antidiuretic hormone increases water reabsorption by the kidney tubules. This decreases urine volume and adds to the fluid in the body. This will also increase blood volume and blood pressure.
• Name the enzyme that stimulates the production of angiotensin II and is produced by the kidneys.
  — Renin, which promotes the production of angiotensin II, is produced by the juxtaglomerular cells.
• Describe two mechanisms by which angiotensin II increases blood pressure.
  — Angiotensin II is a vasoconstrictor, which increases blood pressure. It also stimulates the release of aldosterone, which acts on the kidney tubules to conserve sodium and water. This also increases blood volume and blood pressure.

Characteristics of Urine

- Describe the physical characteristics and chemical composition of urine.
  — Freshly voided urine has a clear yellow color, a specific gravity of 1.001 to 1.035, and a pH between 4.6 and 8.0.
  — Urine is about 95% water and 5% solutes.
- List five abnormal constituents of urine.
  — Abnormal constituents of urine include albumin, glucose, blood cells, ketone bodies, and microbes.

Body Fluids

- State the percentage of body weight that is composed of water.
  — Fluids make up 60% of the adult body weight.
- Identify the major fluid compartments in the body and state the relative amount of fluid in each compartment.
  — Intracellular fluid is the fluid inside the body cells and it accounts for 2/3 of the total body fluid.
  — Extracellular fluid is the fluid outside the body cells and it accounts for 1/3 of the total body fluid.
  — Extracellular fluid is further divided into intravascular fluid (1/5) and interstitial fluid (4/5).
- State the sources of fluid intake and avenues of fluid output and explain how these are regulated to maintain fluid balance.
  — Normally fluid intake equals output. This should be about 2500 ml (2.5 L) per day.
  — Sources of fluid intake are beverages, food, and metabolic water.
  — Avenues of fluid loss are through the kidneys, skin, lungs, and gastrointestinal tract.
  — Fluid intake and fluid loss are regulated by the thirst mechanism and by the water output by the kidneys.
- Identify the major intracellular and extracellular ions and explain how electrolyte balance is regulated.
  — Electrolyte concentrations in the different fluid compartments are different, but they remain relatively constant within each compartment.
  — Sodium (Na^+), chloride (Cl^-), and bicarbonate (HCO_3^-) ions are the predominant ions in the extracellular fluid.
  — Potassium (K^+) and phosphates ($H_2PO_4^-$ and HPO_4^{-2}) are the predominant ions in the intracellular fluid.
  — Aldosterone is the primary regulator of electrolyte concentration through reabsorption of sodium and potassium.
- State the normal pH range of the blood and define the terms acidosis and alkalosis.
  — The normal pH of the blood ranges between 7.35 and 7.45.
  — Deviations below normal are called acidosis and deviations above normal are called alkalosis.
- Describe the three primary mechanisms by which blood pH is regulated.
  — Acid-base balance is maintained through the action of buffers, the lungs, and the kidneys.

LEARNING EXERCISES

Components of the Urinary System

1. What are six functions of the urinary system?

    (a)   (d)

    (b)   (e)

    (c)   (f)

2. Name the four components of the urinary system in the sequence in which urine flows through them.

    (a)   (c)

    (b)   (d)

3. Identify the parts of the kidney by matching the letters from the diagram with the correct structure in the list.

    _____ Major calyx

    _____ Minor calyx

    _____ Renal capsule

    _____ Renal column

    _____ Renal cortex

    _____ Renal papilla

    _____ Renal pelvis

    _____ Renal pyramid

    _____ Ureter

4. Identify the parts of a nephron by matching the letters from the diagram with the correct structure in the list. Draw a box around the renal corpuscle. Draw a circle around the region of the juxtaglomerular apparatus. Use blue to color the portions that are located in the medulla of the kidney.

    _____ Afferent arteriole

    _____ Ascending limb

    _____ Collecting duct

    _____ Descending limb

    _____ Distal convoluted tubule

    _____ Efferent arteriole

    _____ Glomerular capsule

    _____ Glomerulus

    _____ Nephron loop

    _____ Proximal convoluted tubule

5. Write the terms that match the following phrases.

_____ Modified cells in the ascending limb

_____ Modified cells in the afferent arteriole

_____ Enzyme produced by juxtaglomerular cells

_____ Structure that monitors NaCl in the urine

_____ Rate of blood flow through the kidney

_____ Arteries located in the renal sinus

_____ Arteries located in the renal columns

_____ Arteries that pass over the renal pyramids

_____ Branches of the arcuate arteries

_____ Vessel that carries blood to the glomerulus

_____ Capillary network around renal tubules

_____ Location of the interlobar vein

_____ Veins that join to form the renal vein

6. Write the terms that match the following phrases about the ureters, urinary bladder, and urethra.

_____ Transport urine from kidney to urinary bladder

_____ Epithelium in mucosa of ureters

_____ Temporary storage site for urine

_____ Folds in mucosa of urinary bladder

_____ Epithelium in mucosa of urinary bladder

_____ Smooth muscle in wall of urinary bladder

_____ Triangular region in floor of urinary bladder

_____ Muscle type forming internal urethral sphincter

_____ Muscle type forming external urethral sphincter

_____ Transports urine from bladder to outside

_____ Region of the male urethra nearest the bladder

_____ Longest portion of the male urethra

Urine Formation

1. Match each of the three processes involved in urine formation with the correct description of that process.

    _____ Solutes pass from tubular cells into the filtrate   A. glomerular filtration

    _____ Solutes pass from the glomerulus into the capsule   B. tubular reabsorption

    _____ Solutes pass from tubules into peritubular capillaries   C. tubular secretion

2. The following diagram illustrates a glomerulus with the glomerular capsule around it. Representative osmotic and hydrostatic pressures also are indicated. Draw red circles around the pressures that move substances from the glomerulus into the capsule and draw blue circles around the pressures that move substances from the capsule into the glomerulus. Calculate the net filtration pressure.

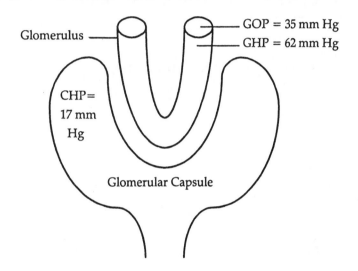

3. Write the terms that match the following phrases about regulation of urine concentration and volume.

    _____ Hormone that increases reabsorption of sodium

    _____ Hormone that increases reabsorption of water

    _____ Hormone that promotes sodium and water loss

    _____ Enzyme produced by juxtaglomerular cells

    _____ Powerful vasoconstrictor

    _____ Act of expelling urine from the urinary bladder

4. Complete the following paragraph about tubular reabsorption and secretion by filling in the correct terms.

1. _____

2. _____

3. _____

4. _____

5. _____

6. _____

7. _____

8. _____

Tubular reabsorption moves substances from the filtrate into the blood and <u>1</u> the volume of urine. Water is reabsorbed by the process of <u>2</u>. Most of the solutes are reabsorbed by <u>3</u> mechanisms. Reabsorption of some solutes is limited by <u>4</u>. When concentration of these solutes exceeds <u>5</u>, the excess appears in the <u>6</u>. Tubular <u>7</u> adds substances to the urine. To help regulate blood pH, <u>8</u> ions are added to the urine and removed from the body by this process.

5. In what two ways does angiotensin II act on the kidneys?

(a)

(b)

Characteristics of Urine

1. Place a check (√) before each of the following statements that is correct.

_____ The color of urine is due to urochrome.

_____ Urine is usually slightly acidic, but may be alkaline.

_____ Normal urine volume is generally about three liters per 24 hours.

_____ High protein diets tend to make urine more alkaline.

_____ The specific gravity of urine is slightly greater than 1.

_____ Solutes make up about 20% of the urine volume.

_____ The predominant solute in urine is urea.

_____ In addition to urea, solutes in urine include glucose and albumin.

2. Write the clinical term that is used to indicate the presence of the following substances in the urine.

_____ White blood cells

_____ Albumin

_____ Glucose

_____ Erythrocytes

Body Fluids

1. List three types of sources for fluid intake. Place an asterisk (*) by the one that normally accounts for the greatest amount of intake.

   (a)

   (b)

   (c)

2. List four avenues of fluid loss and place an asterisk (*) by the one that normally accounts for the greatest amount of loss.

   (a)

   (b)

   (c)

   (d)

3. The following boxes represent the volume of different fluid compartments in the body. Match the letter of each box with the correct name. Also indicate the percent of total body weight that is contained in each compartment.

Compartment	Letter	Percent
Extracellular	_____	_____
Interstitial	_____	_____
Intracellular	_____	_____
Plasma	_____	_____
Solutes	_____	_____
Total fluids	_____	_____

4. Write the terms that match the following phrases about electrolytes in the body.

_____ Predominant cation in extracellular fluid

_____ Predominant anion in extracellular fluid

_____ Predominant cation in intracellular fluid

_____ Predominant anion in intracellular fluid

_____ Primary hormone that regulates electrolytes

5. Write the terms that match the following phrases about acid-base balance in the body.

_____ Normal pH range of the blood

_____ Clinical term for higher than normal pH

_____ Clinical term for lower than normal pH

_____ Primary regulators of blood pH (3)

_____

_____

REVIEW QUESTIONS

1. What is the principal function of the urinary system?

2. List the components of the urinary system in the sequence in which urine flows through them.

3. Describe the location of the kidneys relative to the peritoneum, thoracic vertebrae, and lumbar vertebrae.

4. Identify the regions of the kidney: cortex, medulla, renal column, renal pyramid, capsule, and major and minor calyces.

5. What are the parts of a (a) renal corpuscle and (b) renal tubule?

6. Starting with the glomerular capsule, trace the flow of the filtrate through the kidney to the ureter.

7. What two regions are modified to form the juxtaglomerular apparatus? What does it secrete?

8. The afferent arterioles are branches of what vessels?

9. Where are the ureters located relative to the peritoneum? Where do they enter the urinary bladder?

10. Where is the detrusor muscle located?

11. What is the trigone?

12. What is the difference between the muscle in the internal urethral sphincter and the muscle in the external urethral sphincter?

13. What is micturition?

14. What are the three parts of the male urethra?

15. What are the three processes that are involved in urine formation?

16. How much glomerular filtrate is formed in a 24-hour period?

17. What two components of blood normally are absent from the glomerular filtrate?

18. What two pressures are inversely related to net filtration pressure? In other words, when the two pressures increase, the net filtration pressure decreases.

19. Where does *most* tubular reabsorption take place?

20. What causes glucose to appear in the urine?

21. By what transport mechanism is water reabsorbed?

22. Where in the nephron tubule is water not reabsorbed?

23. What process of urine formation adds substances to the filtrate?

24. If blood volume and/or pressure decreases, what is likely to happen to urine volume? Explain.

25. What three hormones act on the kidney tubules to regulate tubular reabsorption?

26. What is the purpose of renin?

27. What effect does angiotensin II have on the adrenal cortex?

28. How does solute concentration affect the specific gravity of the urine?

29. What terms describe the appearance of the following constituents in the urine: (a) RBCs; (b) glucose; (c) albumin; (d) WBCs?

30. Which fluid compartment has the most volume?

31. In general, what accounts for the most fluid intake? Fluid loss?

32. What is the predominant (a) cation in ECF; (b) cation in ICF; (c) anion in ECF; (d) anion in ICF?

33. What term is used to designate a blood pH of 7.33?

34. How does the urinary system respond if blood pH is too acidic?

CHAPTER QUIZ

1. The functional unit of the kidney is the (a) pyramid; (b) collecting duct; (c) renal corpuscle; (d) nephron.

2. The portion of a nephron that is located in the medulla is the (a) glomerulus; (b) nephron loop of Henle; (c) proximal convoluted tubule; (d) glomerular capsule; (e) distal convoluted tubule.

3. Renin is produced by specialized cells in the (a) medulla; (b) renal pelvis; (c) afferent arteriole; (d) macula densa; (e) glomerulus.

4. The arteries that are located in the renal columns are the (a) interlobar arteries; (b) arcuate arteries; (c) segmental arteries; (d) interlobular arteries; (e) renal arteries.

5. Name the following:

   _____   Smooth muscle in the wall of the urinary bladder

   _____   Triangular region in the floor of the urinary bladder

   _____   Voluntary sphincter of the urethra

   _____   Proximal or first portion of the male urethra

6. The following represents a nephron tubule and a blood capillary. Draw arrows to indicate whether substances move from the capillary into the tubule or from the tubule into the capillary in each of the three steps in urine formation.

	Glomerular Filtration	Tubular Reabsorption	Tubular Secretion
Capillary			
Tubule			

7. Indicate whether each of the following factors increases or decreases the volume of urine.

   _____   Decreased capillary osmotic pressure

   _____   Increased tubular reabsorption of water

   _____   Decreased secretion of ADH

   _____   Increased secretion of aldosterone

   _____   Increased secretion of renin

8. Assume an adult male weighs 80 kg.

   How many liters of water are in his body?

How many liters of intracellular fluid are there?

How many liters of interstitial fluid are there?

9. Which of the following is the primary extracellular cation? (a) sodium; (b) chloride; (c) potassium; (d) phosphate; (e) bicarbonate

10. Which of the following blood pH values represents acidosis? (a) 7.5; (b) 7.4; (c) 7.3; (d) none of the above; (e) all of the above

USING CLINICAL KNOWLEDGE

1. Match the definitions on the left with the correct term from the column on the right by placing the corresponding letter in the space before the definition. Not all terms will be used.

_____ Plasma	A. Acidosis
_____ Functional unit of the kidney	B. Alkalosis
_____ Increased amounts of nitrogenous waste products in the blood	C. Azotemia
	D. Cystoscopy
_____ Producing small amounts of urine	E. Diuretic
_____ Crushing of a calculus in kidney or bladder	F. Enuresis
_____ May be caused by hyperventilation	G. Glomerulus
_____ Associated with defective uric acid metabolism	H. Gout
_____ Increases the production of urine	I. Intracellular fluid
_____ Visual examination of the urinary bladder	J. Intravascular fluid
_____ Involuntary emission of urine; bedwetting	K. Lithotripsy
	L. Nephron
	M. Oliguria

2. Write the meaning of the following abbreviations.

_____   BUN

_____   ARF

_____   GFR

_____   TUR

_____   UTI

3. Spelling is important in scientific and medical applications because only one or two incorrect letters may change the meaning. Circle the correctly spelled word for each of the following pairs.

detrusor	detrussor
macula densa	macula denca
triagone	trigone
natriuretic	natrietic
albuminuria	albuminaria

4. Write the meaning of the underlined portion of each word on the line preceding the word.

_____   <u>nephr</u>optosis

_____   <u>cyst</u>itis

_____   <u>pyelo</u>lithotomy

_____ nephro<u>lithi</u>asis

_____ <u>azo</u>temia

_____ <u>noc</u>turia

_____ <u>peri</u>tubular

_____ nephro<u>pexy</u>

_____ uretero<u>rrhaphy</u>

_____ <u>juxta</u>glomerular

5. Rhea Knull experiences excessive urination during the night. What is the clinical term for this condition?

6. Sarah has diabetes mellitus which she finds difficult to control. On her last visit to her doctor, she had ketosis and a below normal blood pH. She also exhibited an increased respiratory rate.

    a. What is ketosis?

    b. What acid/base imbalance does she have?

    c. Is this a respiratory or metabolic imbalance?

    d. Why is the respiratory rate increased?

FUN AND GAMES

Each of the puzzles below consists of a series of clues for which the answers add up to solve the puzzle. The individual clues are followed by a series of blanks with numbers. When you have determined the answer to a clue, transfer the letters to the correspondingly numbered spaces for the total or final answer. If there is no number under a blank, that letter does not appear in the final answer.

Clues   *Answers*

Vessel leading into the glomerulus   __ __ __ __ __ __ __ __   __ __ __ __ __ __ __ __ __
                                  16 11 11 5 10 5 20 17   9 6 14 5 10 12 19 8 5

Reduced urine output   __ __ __ __ __ __ __ __
                                                       3 13 18 1 7 15 12 9

Normal fluid intake is 2500 _____   __ __
                                                                   4 2

TOTAL: First process in urine formation

__ __ __ __ __ __ __ __ __ __ __ __ __ __ __ __ __ __ __ __
1 2 3 4 5 6 7 8 9 10 11 12 13 14 15 16 17 18 19 20

Convoluted tubule preceding nephron loop   __ __ __ __ __ __ __
                                                          17 11 8 3 9 14 7

Fluid portion of blood   __ __ __ __ __ __
                                                          18 13 5 24 9 16

Prefix meaning near to   __ __ __ __ __
                                                           1 23 3 22 16

Root meaning without an opening   __ __ __ __ __ __
                                                          19 4 15 10 24 21

Folds in bladder wall   __ __ __ __ __
                                                           20 2 6 21 10

Twenty-first letter of the alphabet   __
                                                                12

TOTAL: Structure that monitors blood flow and secretes renin

__ __
1 2 3 4 5 6 7 8 9 10 11 12 13 14 15 16 17 18 19 20 21 22 23 24

Outer region of kidney   __ __ __ __ __
                                                           6 13 3 7 2

Vessel leading away from glomerulus   __ __ __ __ __ __ __ __ __ __ __ __ __ __ __
                                   1 14 14 7 4 1 3 5 13 3 1 4 17 8 1

Inner region of kidney   __ __ __ __ __ __
                                                           7 18 10 9 15 12

Indentation on medial side of kidney   __ __ __
                                                            17 11 16

TOTAL: Makes up 20% of the adult body weight

__ __ __ __ __ __ __ __ __ __ __ __ __ __ __ __ __ __
1 2 3 4 5 6 7 8 9 10 11 12 13 14 15 16 17 18

Reproductive System

KEY TERMS

Gametes
Gonads
Oogenesis
Ovarian cycle
Ovarian follicle
Spermatogenesis
Spermiogenesis
Uterine cycle

BUILDING VOCABULARY

andr-
balan-
colpo-
crypt-
ejacul-
episi-
fimb-
follic-
genit-
gynec-
hyster-
labi-
lapar-
mamm-
meno-
metr-
oo-
oophor-
orch-
ov-
prostat-
-rrhagia
salping-
-spadias

CLINICAL TERMS

Amenorrhea
Anorchism
Azoospermia
Circumcision
Coitus
Curettage
Dysmenorrhea
Endometriosis
Episiotomy
Hysterectomy
Mittelschmerz
Oligospermia
Oophorectomy
Orchidectomy
Phimosis
Prostatitis
Salpingectomy
Spermicide
Vaginoplasty
Vasectomy

CLINICAL ABBREVIATIONS

BPH
Cx
D&C
IUD
LMP
Pap
PID
PMS
PSA
STD
TAH
TURP
VD

OUTLINE/OBJECTIVES

Male Reproductive System

- Distinguish between the primary and secondary reproductive organs.
  — Primary, or essential, reproductive organs are the gonads. In the male, the gonads are the testes and in the female they are the ovaries.
  — Secondary reproductive organs include all other components of the reproductive system, including the ducts, glands, and accessory organs.
- Describe the location and structure of each component of the male reproductive system.
  — The testes, located in the scrotum, are surrounded by the tunica albuginea, which extends inward to divide the organ into lobules. Each lobule contains seminiferous tubules and interstitial cells. Sperm are produced in the seminiferous tubules and the interstitial cells produce testosterone.
  — The epididymis is a convoluted tube on the margin of the testis. Sperm mature and become fertile in the epididymis.
  — The ductus deferens begins at the epididymis and extends to the ejaculatory duct posterior to the urinary bladder.
  — The ejaculatory duct is a short passageway that is formed when the ductus deferens and the duct from the seminal vesicles join. It penetrates the prostate gland and empties into the urethra.
  — The male urethra is a passageway for sperm, fluids from the reproductive system, and urine. It is divided into the prostatic urethra, membranous urethra, and penile urethra.
  — Seminal vesicles are paired, saccular glands posterior to the urinary bladder. Secretion from these glands contributes over 60% of the volume of seminal fluid and contains fructose, prostaglandins, and coagulation proteins.
  — The prostate is a firm dense gland located inferior to the urinary bladder; it encircles the proximal part of the urethra. Prostatic secretions are alkaline and enhance motility of sperm.
  — The bulbourethral glands are located near the base of the penis and secrete a viscous alkaline fluid, which neutralizes acidity of vagina and provides lubrication during intercourse.
  — Seminal fluid or semen is a mixture of sperm cells and the secretions of the accessory glands. Emission is the discharge of semen into the urethra; ejaculation is the forceful expulsion of semen from the urethra.
  — The penis consists of three columns of erectile tissue. The two dorsal columns are the corpora cavernosa and the ventral column is the corpus spongiosum. The root of the penis attaches it to the pubic arch, the body is the visible portion, and the glans penis is the expanded tip of corpus spongiosum. The urethra extends through the entire length of the penis.
- Draw and label a diagram or flow chart that illustrates spermatogenesis and describe the process by which spermatids become mature sperm.
  — Spermatogenesis, which begins at puberty, is the process by which spermatids are formed. Spermatogonia become primary spermatocytes and each spermatocyte produces four spermatids by meiosis.
  — Spermiogenesis changes spermatids into mature spermatozoa, each with a head, midpiece, and tail. The head contains the nucleus, the midpiece contains mitochondria, and the tail is a flagellum for movement.
- Trace the pathway of sperm from the testes to the outside of the body.
  — Spermatozoa are produced in the seminiferous tubules of the testes then pass through the duct system to reach the outside.
  — From the seminiferous tubules, the sperm enter the epididymis, then the ductus deferens to the ejaculatory duct and into the urethra.
- Outline the physiologic events in the male sexual response.

- — The male sexual response includes erection and orgasm accompanied by ejaculation of semen.
- — Orgasm is followed by a variable time period during which it is not possible to achieve another erection.
- Describe the role of GnRH, FSH, LH, and testosterone in male reproductive functions.
  - — At puberty, the hypothalamus secretes GnRH, which stimulates the anterior pituitary to secrete FSH and LH.
  - — FSH stimulates the seminiferous tubules and spermatogenesis.
  - — LH stimulates the interstitial cells and the production of testosterone.
  - — Testosterone from the interstitial cells stimulates the development of the secondary sex characteristics and spermatogenesis.

Female Reproductive System

- Describe the location and structure of each component of the female reproductive system, including the mammary glands.
  - — The female gonads are the ovaries, which are located on each side of the uterus in the pelvic cavity. They are covered with simple cuboidal epithelium around the tunica albuginea. Numerous ovarian follicles make the cortex appear granular; the medulla is connective tissue with vessels and nerves.
  - — The uterine tubes, also called fallopian tubes or oviducts, extend laterally from each side of the uterus. The end of the uterine tube near the ovary expands to form the infundibulum. Fingerlike projections, called fimbriae, extend from the infundibulum.
  - — The uterus consists of a fundus, body, and cervix. The broad ligament is a fold of peritoneum that extends laterally from the uterus to the pelvic wall. The fundus and body of the uterus are normally anteflexed over the superior surface of the urinary bladder. The internal os is the opening from the body into the cervix; the external os is the opening from the cervix into the vagina. Visceral peritoneum forms the perimetrium, the outer layer of the uterine wall; smooth muscle makes up the thick myometrium; and the endometrium is mucous membrane. The endometrium is separated into a deeper stratum basale and superficial stratum functionale.
  - — The vagina extends from the cervix to the exterior. It serves as a passageway for menstrual flow, receives the erect penis during intercourse, and is the birth canal during the birth of a baby.
  - — Collectively, the female external genitalia are referred to as the vulva or pudendum. This includes the labia majora, mons pubis, labia minora, clitoris, and accessory glands. The area between the two labia minora is the vestibule. The clitoris (erectile tissue) is at the anterior end of the vestibule. Paraurethral and greater vestibular glands, accessory glands of the female reproductive tract, open into the vestibule. The urethra and vagina also open into the vestibule.
  - — The mammary glands, located within the breast, consist of lobules of glandular units that produce milk. Lactiferous ducts transport the milk to the nipple. Cords of connective tissue, called suspensory ligaments, help support the breast. Estrogen and progesterone stimulate the development of glandular tissue and ducts in the breast. Prolactin stimulates the production of milk. Oxytocin causes the ejection of the milk from the breast.
- Draw and label a diagram or flow chart that illustrates oogenesis.
  - — Oogenesis begins in prenatal development with the formation of the primary oocyte. Division ceases in this stage and the oocytes remain dormant until puberty.
  - — Beginning at puberty, each month, a primary oocyte resumes meiosis and produces a secondary oocyte and a polar body. Division again halts.
  - — If a sperm penetrates the oocyte, meiosis resumes and a mature egg and another polar body

are produced.

— Oogenesis differs from spermatogenesis in that each primary oocyte produces one ovum and three nonfunctional polar bodies; each primary spermatocyte produces four spermatids. Beginning at puberty, spermatogenesis is a continuous process; oogenesis occurs in monthly cycles. Spermatogenesis doesn't begin until puberty; oogenesis begins in prenatal development.

- Describe the development of ovarian follicles as they progress from primordial follicles to primary follicles, secondary follicles, vesicular follicles, corpus luteum, and finally, the corpus albicans.
  — An ovarian follicle consists of an oocyte with one or more layers of cells surrounding it.
  — Primordial follicles, each with a primary oocyte surrounded by a single layer of cells, are the follicles present at birth.
  — At puberty the primordial follicles begin to grow and become secondary follicles, and some mature and become vesicular follicles.
  — Vesicular follicles rupture at ovulation and release their secondary oocyte.
  — Follicles develop under the influence of FSH; follicle cells produce estrogen.
  — After ovulation, the follicle cells are transformed into a corpus luteum that produces progesterone. The corpus luteum degenerates into a corpus albicans

- Outline the physiologic events in the female sexual response.
  — The female sexual response includes erection and orgasm, but there is no ejaculation.
  — A woman may become pregnant without having an orgasm.

- Describe the roles of GnRH, FSH, LH, estrogen, and progesterone in female reproductive functions.
  — GnRH, FSH, LH, estrogen, and progesterone interact to create the ovarian and uterine cycles.

- Describe what happens in each phase of the ovarian and uterine cycles, when each phase occurs, and how the cycles interact.
  — The monthly ovarian cycle begins with the follicle development during the follicular phase, continues with ovulation during the ovulatory phase, and concludes with the development and regression of the corpus luteum during the luteal phase.
  — The follicle develops under the influence of FSH. As the follicle matures, it secretes increasing amounts of estrogen. At ovulation, the estrogen level falls, then the corpus luteum, under the influence of LH, begins secreting progesterone.
  — The uterine cycle takes place simultaneously with the ovarian cycle.
  — The uterine cycle begins with menstruation during the menstrual phase, continues with repair of the endometrium during the proliferative phase, and ends with the growth of glands and blood vessels during the secretory phase.
  — The menstrual phase is the result of decreased amounts of progesterone and estrogen from the corpus luteum; estrogen from developing follicles is responsible for the proliferative phase, and progesterone from the corpus luteum is responsible for the secretory phase.
  — Menarche is the first menstrual flow; menopause is the time when the monthly ovarian and uterine cycles cease.

LEARNING EXERCISES

Male Reproductive System

1. Identify the parts of the male reproductive system by matching the letters from the diagram with the correct structure in the list.

    _____   Bulbourethral gland

    _____   Corpus cavernosum

    _____   Corpus spongiosum

    _____   Ductus deferens

    _____   Ejaculatory duct

    _____   Epididymis

    _____   Glans penis

    _____   Prostate

    _____   Scrotum

    _____   Symphysis pubis

    _____   Testicle

    _____   Urethra (2 places)

    _____

    _____   Urinary bladder

2. Number the following structures in the correct sequence, from 1 to 10, to trace the pathway of sperm from the seminiferous tubule to the exterior. Start with #1 for the seminiferous tubule.

    _____   Ductus deferens   _____   Penile urethra

    _____   Efferent ducts   _____   Prostatic urethra

    _____   Ejaculatory duct   _____   Rete testis

    _____   Epididymis   _____   Seminiferous tubules

    _____   Membranous urethra   _____   Straight tubules

3. Write the terms that match the following phrases about the male reproductive system.

    _____   Male gonad

    _____   Male gamete

    _____   Pouch of skin that contains the male gonad

    _____   Smooth muscle in subcutaneous tissue of scrotum

    _____   Skeletal muscle fibers in the spermatic cord

_____ Fibrous connective tissue capsule of the testes

_____ Specific location of spermatogenesis

_____ Cells that produce male sex hormones

_____ Maturation of spermatids into spermatozoa

_____ Region of spermatozoa that contains mitochondria

_____ Number of chromosomes in a spermatid

_____ Cells that nourish developing spermatids

4. Match each of the following phrases with the accessory gland to which it pertains.

_____ Product secreted into the penile urethra

_____ Encircles the proximal portion of the urethra

_____ Located posterior to the urinary bladder

_____ Secretion accounts for 60% of the seminal fluid

_____ Located near the base of the penis

_____ Smallest of the accessory glands

_____ Secretion has a high fructose content

A. seminal vesicles

B. prostate

C. bulbourethral gland

5. Complete the following paragraph about the male sexual response by filling in the correct terms.

1. _____

2. _____

3. _____

4. _____

5. _____

6. _____

7. _____

8. _____

9. _____

10. _____

11. _____

During sexual stimulation 1 impulses dilate the 2 and constrict the 3 of the penis. This causes the spaces in the erectile tissue to fill with blood and the penis enlarges and becomes rigid. This is called 4. With continued stimulation, these reflexes become more intense until they prompt a surge of 5 impulses to the genital organs. These impulses cause the forceful discharge of semen into the urethra. This is called 6. 7, the forceful expulsion of semen to the exterior, immediately follows. The muscular contractions that result in the expulsion of semen are accompanied by feelings of pleasure, 8 heart rate, 9 blood pressure, and 10. Collectively, these physiological responses are referred to as 11.

6. Write the terms that match the following phrases about the hormones that control male reproductive functions.

_____	Hypothalamic hormone that initiates puberty
_____	Hormone from the interstitial cells
_____	Hormone that stimulates the interstitial cells
_____	Collective term for male sex hormones
_____	With testosterone it stimulates spermatogenesis
_____	Anterior pituitary hormones that act on testes (2)
_____	
_____	Source of testosterone before birth
_____	Functions of testosterone (2)
_____	

Female Reproductive System

1. Identify the parts of the female reproductive system by matching the letters from the diagram with the correct structure in the list.

_____ Cervix

_____ Clitoris

_____ Infundibulum

_____ Mons pubis

_____ Ovary

_____ Rectum

_____ Symphysis pubis

_____ Urethra

_____ Urinary bladder

_____ Uterine tube

_____ Uterus

_____ Vagina

2. Write the terms that match the following phrases about the internal female reproductive system.

_____	Female gonad
_____	Stage of oogenesis present at birth
_____	Stage of oogenesis that is ovulated each month

_____ Clear glycoprotein membrane around an oocyte

_____ Cells around oocyte at ovulation

_____ Develops from follicle after ovulation

_____ Fingerlike extensions of the uterine tubes

_____ Opening from the cervix into the vagina

_____ Largest ligament that stabilizes the uterus

_____ Muscular layer of the uterus

_____ Endometrial region shed during menstruation

_____ Mucous membrane covering vaginal orifice

3. Identify the structures associated with the ovary and uterine tube by matching the letters from the diagram with the correct item in the list.

_____ Antrum

_____ Corpus albicans

_____ Corpus luteum

_____ Fimbriae

_____ Infundibulum

_____ Primary follicle

_____ Secondary follicle

_____ Secondary oocyte

_____ Uterine tube

_____ Vesicular follicle

4. Write the terms that match the following phrases about the female external genitalia.

_____ Collective term for female external genitalia

_____ Fat-filled folds of skin that enclose the genitalia

_____ Mound of fat that overlies the symphysis pubis

_____ Area between the two labia minora

_____ Female structure homologous to male penis

_____ Glands adjacent to the urethral orifice

_____ Glands adjacent to the vaginal orifice

5. Write T before the true statements and F before the false statements about the female sexual response.

_____ The female sexual response consists of erection and orgasm.

_____ Sympathetic responses to sexual stimuli produce increased blood flow to erectile tissue.

_____ Sympathetic responses produce rhythmic contractions of the uterus and pelvic floor, accompanied by feelings of intense pleasure.

6. Match the following statements and phrases with the correct hormone. Some may have more than one correct response. Give all correct answers.

_____ Starts the events of puberty

_____ Levels increase after menopause

_____ Secreted by the hypothalamus

_____ Secreted by the anterior pituitary

_____ Triggers ovulation

_____ Secreted by the corpus luteum

_____ Secreted by cells of the ovarian follicle

_____ Stimulates secretory phase of uterine cycle

_____ Stimulates proliferative phase of uterine cycle

_____ Stimulates development of the corpus luteum

_____ Stimulates development of glandular tissue in the breast

_____ Stimulates development of the duct system in the breast

_____ Causes an accumulation of adipose tissue in the breast

_____ Stimulates growth of ovarian follicles

_____ Levels decrease after menopause

A. gonadotropin-releasing hormone

B. follicle-stimulating hormone

C. luteinizing hormone

D. estrogen

E. progesterone

7. Complete the following statements by using the words *increases* or *decreases*.

As ovarian follicles grow in response to FSH, estrogen secretion _____.

Blood estrogen level _____ during days 6-13 of the menstrual cycle.

After ovulation, progesterone secretion _____.

An increasing level of progesterone _____ LH secretion.

The menstrual phase of the uterine cycle is caused by _____ in progesterone levels.

8. Write the terms that match the following phrases about the breast.

_____ Circular pigmented area around the nipple

_____ Bands of connective tissue that support the breast

_____ Collects the milk from the glandular units

_____ Dilated region of duct that is a reservoir for milk

_____ Hormone that stimulates milk production

_____ Hormone that causes ejection of milk from glands

REVIEW QUESTIONS

1. What organs are primary reproductive organs and what is their function?

2. Identify the parts of the male reproductive system: testis, scrotum, epididymis, ductus deferens, prostate, prostatic urethra, ejaculatory duct, membranous urethra, bulbourethral gland, spongy urethra, and penis.

3. Where are the male gonads located early in their development? Where are they normally located at birth?

4. Where are the seminiferous tubules located and what is their function?

5. How many chromosomes are in a (a) spermatogonium; (b) primary spermatocyte; (c) secondary spermatocyte; (d) spermatid; (e) spermatozoa?

6. In mature spermatozoa, what is contained in the (a) acrosome; (b) head; (c) midpiece?

7. What duct do the sperm enter when they leave the (a) epididymis; (b) ejaculatory duct?

8. Which accessory gland makes the largest contribution to the seminal fluid? Where are these glands located?

9. In reference to seminal fluid, what is meant by the term "emission"?

10. What erectile tissue surrounds the urethra in the penis?

11. What effects do FSH and LH have on the testes?

12. Identify the parts of the female reproductive system: ovary, uterus, uterine tubes, mons pubis, cervix, vagina, urethra, labia majora, labia minora, clitoris, and mons pubis.

13. What type of follicles are in the ovarian cortex of a normal 5-year-old girl?

14. How many secondary oocytes are produced from each primary oocyte? How does this compare with the number of secondary spermatocytes that are produced from each primary spermatocyte?

15. What two structures (or layers) surround the secondary oocyte in a vesicular follicle?

16. What stage of meiosis is released at the time of ovulation?

17. What portion of the uterine tubes is closest to the ovaries?

18. What portion of the uterus is between the internal os and the external os?

19. What specific portion of the uterine wall is sloughed off during menstruation?

20. What is the purpose of the vagina? Where does it open to the exterior?

21. Where are the greater vestibular glands located and what is their purpose?

22. What hormone is increasing during the follicular phase of the ovarian cycle?

23. What phase of the uterine cycle corresponds to the luteal phase of the ovarian cycle? What hormones are increasing during this period?

24. What effects do estrogen and progesterone have on the structure of the mammary glands?

25. How does the posterior pituitary affect the mammary glands?

CHAPTER QUIZ

1. Which of the following best describes a difference between spermatogenesis and oogenesis? (a) a primary spermatocyte produces four spermatids but a primary oocyte produces only two ova; (b) primary spermatocytes all develop after puberty but primary oocytes all develop before birth; (c) secondary spermatocytes have 46 chromosomes but secondary oocytes have only 23; (d) LH stimulates spermatogenesis but FSH stimulates oogenesis.

2. Arrange the given ducts in the correct sequence for the passage of sperm: (1) ejaculatory duct; (2) epididymis; (3) urethra; (4) ductus deferens; (5) efferent duct.
   (a) 2, 4, 1, 3, 5
   (b) 4, 5, 2, 1, 3
   (c) 5, 2, 4, 3, 1
   (d) 5, 2, 4, 1, 3

3. Indicate whether each of the following phrases best describes the seminal vesicles (S), the prostate (P), or the bulbourethral glands (B).

   _____   Encircles the urethra

   _____   Contributes about 60% of the seminal fluid volume

   _____   Empties into the penile urethra

   _____   Secretion is thin and milky-colored

   _____   Empties into the ejaculatory duct

4. Place an X before the following phrases that describe the corpus spongiosum.

   _____   Erectile tissue   _____   Makes up the glans penis

   _____   Dorsal   _____   Two columns

   _____   Encircles the urethra

5. Match the following hormones with their actions. There is only one *best* response for each action.

   _____   Stimulates the interstitial cells   A. FSH

   _____   Hormone from the hypothalamus   B. GnRH

   _____   Secreted by the ovary during the follicular phase   C. LH

   _____   Stimulates production of testosterone   D. estrogen

   _____   Promotes glandular secretion in the endometrium   E. progesterone

   _____   Stimulates secretion of FSH   F. testosterone

   _____   Promotes repair of uterine lining after menstruation

   _____   Stimulates the seminiferous tubules

   _____   Promotes male secondary sex characteristics

   _____   With testosterone, stimulates spermatogenesis

6. What noncellular layer surrounds the oocyte at the time of ovulation? (a) corona radiata; (b) zona pellucida; (c) granulosa; (d) antrum

7. The portion of the uterine wall that changes during the uterine cycle is the (a) myometrium; (b) perimetrium; (c) stratum basale; (d) stratum functionale.

8. At what time in the ovarian cycle is the secretion of LH at a maximum?

9. Which one of the following is *not* true about the vulva? (a) labia majora have an abundance of adipose; (b) labia minora form the prepuce over the clitoris; (c) the clitoris is the most anterior structure in the vestibule; (d) the opening for the vagina is anterior to the urethra

10. What effect does each of the following hormones have on the mammary glands?

Estrogen

Progesterone

Prolactin

Oxytocin

USING CLINICAL KNOWLEDGE

1. Match the definitions on the left with the correct term from the column on the right by placing the corresponding letter in the space before the definition. Not all terms will be used.

_____ Sex cells; sperm and ova	A. Coitus
_____ Combination estrogen and progestin oral contraceptive that most closely resembles hormone levels during a normal monthly cycle	B. Curettage
	C. Gametes
_____ Abdominal pain that may occur at time of ovulation	D. Gonads
	E. Mittelschmerz
_____ Surgical removal of a testis	F. Monophasic
_____ Low sperm count	G. Oligospermia
_____ Primary reproductive organs	H. Orchidectomy
_____ Synthetic progesterone	I. Phimosis
_____ Surgical removal of a uterine tube	J. Progestin
_____ Removal of a growth or other matter from the uterus by scraping or suction	K. Salpingectomy
_____ Sexual intercourse between a man and a woman	L. Triphasic

2. Write the meaning of the following abbreviations.

_____ PMS

_____ STD

_____ VD

_____ IUD

_____ PID

3. Spelling is important in scientific and medical applications because only one or two incorrect letters may change the meaning. Circle the correctly spelled word for each of the following pairs.

menarche	menarch
primodial	primordial
pudenum	pudendum
hysterectomy	histerectomy
prostate	prostrate
semineferous	seminiferous
epididymis	epidydimis
mammry	mammary
antiflexed	anteflexed
perimetrium	parametrium

4. Write the meaning of the underlined portion of each word on the line preceding the word.

_____ <u>men</u>opause

_____ <u>fimbri</u>ae

_____ <u>colp</u>oscopy

_____ lap<u>aro</u>scopy

_____ <u>epi</u>siotomy

_____ crypt<u>orchid</u>ism

_____ <u>crypt</u>orchidism

_____ <u>balan</u>itis

_____ hypo<u>spad</u>ias

_____ <u>ejacul</u>ation

5. James had an enlarged prostate gland, and his doctor ordered a blood test for PSA. It was determined that he had benign prostatic hypertrophy and treatment included a TURP.

   a. What is PSA?

   b. What is another term for benign prostatic hypertrophy?

   c. What is TURP?

6. Carol, who is 23, is athletic and trains regularly for running marathons. Now she is concerned because it has been three months since her last menstrual period and she is not pregnant. What is the clinical term for her condition?

FUN AND GAMES

Some of the following statements are true and others are false. If the statement is true, circle the letter in the true column. If the statement is false, circle the letter in the false column. When you have finished, unscramble the circled letters in the true column to form a word that indicates the subject of this chapter. Do the same for the letters in the false column to find a second related word.

True	*False*	*Statements*
N	A	Sperm are formed within the seminiferous tubules of the testes.
E	N	Sustentacular cells secrete testosterone.
O	U	The mitochondria of the sperm are located in the tailpiece where they provide energy for the flagellum.
R	C	Sperm production is a continuous process that begins at puberty and continues throughout the life of a male.
D	T	The urethra is longer in males than in females.
C	I	Untreated cryptorchidism results in male sterility.
S	O	Fluid from the prostate contains fructose and makes up about 60% of the semen.
M	I	The male urethra is surrounded by corpus cavernosum in the penis.
O	B	Erection of the penis results when the venous sinuses in the erectile tissue become engorged with blood.
W	Y	The forceful discharge of semen into the urethra is called ejaculation.
E	D	FSH stimulates seminiferous tubules in males and ovarian follicles in females.
G	T	Four secondary oocytes develop from each oogonium during meiosis.
O	J	The corpus luteum secretes estrogen in addition to progesterone.
K	N	The oviduct is continuous with the ovary at one end and the uterus at the other.
T	L	The uterus normally is anteflexed over the superior surface of the urinary bladder.
P	S	The stratum basale of the endometrium functions to rebuild the stratum functionale after menstruation.
I	U	The thickest portion of the uterine wall is the myometrium.
A	T	The urethra and vagina open into a region called the vulva.
U	B	Parasympathetic responses to sexual stimuli produce increased blood flow to the clitoris.
D	C	The follicular phase of the ovarian cycle corresponds to the secretory phase of the uterine cycle.
G	I	Spermatozoa and ova are approximately the same size.
R	L	The hypothalamus secretes releasing factors that regulate, to some extent, the secretion of gonadotropic hormones from the pituitary gland.

True Letters _____   Word _____

False Letters _____   Word _____

Development

KEY TERMS

Amnion
Chorion
Cleavage
Embryonic period
Fetal period
Implantation
Parturition
Preembryonic period
Zygote

BUILDING VOCABULARY

amnio-
-blast
-cente
cleav-
contra-
cyesi-
cyst-
galacto-
gravid-
morpho-
morul-
nat-
nulli-
oxy-
para-
partur-
sen-
-toc-
umbil-
zyg-

CLINICAL TERMS

Abruptio placentae
Amniocentesis
Apgar score
Cesarean section
Dystocia
Eclampsia
Ectopic pregnancy
Episiotomy
Eutocia
Lochia
Miscarriage
Multipara
Neonate
Nullipara
Pelvimetry
Placenta previa
Preeclampsia
Stillbirth
Teratogen

CLINICAL ABBREVIATIONS

C-section
CVS
EDC
EDD
EFM
FAS
FHR
GYN
LMP
NB
OB
SAB
SIDS
TAB

OUTLINE/OBJECTIVES

Fertilization

- Describe the events in the process of fertilization, state where it normally occurs, and name the cell that is formed as a result of fertilization.
  - Prenatal development is the period from fertilization to birth. Postnatal development is the period from birth to death.
  - As the sperm move through the female reproductive tract, the acrosome membrane weakens. This is called capacitation.
  - The process of fertilization begins when a single sperm penetrates the cell membrane of a secondary oocyte. This stimulates completion of the second meiotic division, which produces a second polar body and an ovum. The nuclear membranes of the male and female pronuclei degenerate and the two nuclei fuse.
  - The fertilized egg, which has a full complement of 46 chromosomes, is called a zygote.
  - Fertilization normally takes place in the uterine tube.
- Name the three divisions of prenatal development and state the period of time for each one.
  - Prenatal development consists of a preembryonic period (2 weeks), embryonic period (6 weeks), and fetal period (30 weeks).

Preembryonic Period (2 weeks)

- Describe three significant developments that take place during the preembryonic period.
  - Cleavage is a rapid series of mitotic cell divisions after fertilization. The cells that result are blastomeres.
  - A solid ball of blastomeres is a morula. A cavity forms inside the morula and it becomes a blastocyst.
  - The cavity inside the blastocyst is the blastocele and the cells around the outside are the trophoblast. A cluster of cells on one side is the inner cell mass and represents the future embryo.
  - Implantation occurs as endometrial tissue grows around the blastocyst. The entire process takes about 7 days.
  - The trophoblast cells secrete human chorionic gonadotropin, which acts like LH to maintain the corpus luteum. Since the corpus luteum continues to secrete progesterone, the uterine lining is maintained and menstruation is inhibited.
  - The three primary germ layers develop while implantation is taking place.
  - The primary germ layers are ectoderm, mesoderm, and endoderm.

Embryonic Development (6 weeks)

- Describe three significant developments that take place during the embryonic period.
  - The amnion, chorion, yolk sac, and allantois are membranes that form outside the embryo and are called extraembryonic membranes.
  - The extraembryonic membranes function in protection, nutrition, and excretion for the embryo.
  - The amnion forms from the outer layer of the inner cell mass. It forms a fluid-filled sac that surrounds the growing embryo. It helps maintain constant temperature and pressure around the embryo, and provides for symmetrical development and movement.
  - The chorion develops from the trophoblast and contributes to the formation of the placenta.

- The yolk sac develops from the endoderm side of the embryonic disk and produces the primordial germ cells.
- The allantois develops from the yolk sac and contributes to the formation of the umbilical arteries and vein.
- The placenta develops from the endometrium of the uterus and the chorion of the embryo.
- Chorionic villi grow into the endometrium, and blood-filled lacunae from the endometrium surround the villi.
- Nutrients and oxygen diffuse from the mother's blood in the lacunae into the blood vessels in the chorionic villi. Waste materials diffuse in the opposite direction.
- The placenta functions as a temporary endocrine gland for the mother and produces estrogen and progesterone.
- All body organs develop from the ectoderm, mesoderm, and endoderm that are formed during the preembryonic period.
- All organ systems are formed by the end of the embryonic period.
- List five derivatives from each of the primary germ layers.
  - Ectoderm: epidermis of the skin, hair, nails, skin glands, lens of the eye, enamel of the teeth, all nervous tissue, adrenal medulla, sense organ receptor cells, linings of the oral and nasal cavities, vagina, and anal canal.
  - Mesoderm: dermis of the skin; skeletal, smooth, cardiac muscle; connective tissue including cartilage and bone; epithelium of serous membranes; epithelium of joint cavities; epithelium of blood vessels, kidneys and ureters; adrenal cortex; epithelium of gonads and reproductive ducts.
  - Endoderm: epithelial lining of digestive tract; epithelium of the liver and pancreas; epithelium of urinary bladder and urethra; epithelium of the respiratory tract; and thyroid, parathyroid, and thymus glands.

Fetal Development (30 weeks)

- State the two fundamental processes that take place during fetal development.
  - The fetal period is one of growth and maturation of the organ systems that form during the embryonic period.
- Name, describe the location, and state the function of five structures that are unique in the circulatory pattern of the fetus.
  - Since the lungs and liver are nonfunctional during the fetal period, special structures in the circulatory pathway allow blood to bypass these organs. Other vessels take blood to and from the placenta for gaseous exchange.
  - Two umbilical arteries carry fetal blood to the placenta and one umbilical vein returns the oxygenated blood to fetal circulation. The ductus venosus carries blood from the umbilical vein to the inferior vena cava and bypasses the liver. The foramen ovale, in the interatrial septum, and the ductus arteriosus, between the pulmonary trunk and descending aorta, allow blood to bypass the lungs.

Parturition and Lactation

- Describe the roles of the hypothalamus, estrogen, progesterone, oxytocin, and prostaglandins in promoting labor.
  - Gestation period is the time from fertilization to birth; it is the time of pregnancy. It normally lasts for 266 days from fertilization, or 280 days from the beginning of the last menstrual period.
  - Parturition refers to the birth of a baby and labor is the process by which forceful contractions expel the fetus from the uterus.

— Near the end of gestation, estrogen levels increase and progesterone starts to decrease. This removes progesterone's inhibitory effects on the uterus. Estrogen also sensitizes oxytocin receptors. Pressure of the baby's head on the cervix signals the hypothalamus to secrete oxytocin and this, with prostaglandins, stimulates uterine contractions.

- Describe the three stages of labor.
  — The dilation stage of labor begins with the onset of true labor and lasts until the cervix is fully dilated. The expulsion stage lasts from full cervical dilation until delivery of the fetus. The final phase is the placental stage when the placenta and extraembryonic membranes are expelled.

- Describe the changes that take place in the baby's respiratory system and circulatory pathway at birth or soon after birth.
  — When the umbilical cord is cut, the baby's oxygen supply from the mother is terminated. Changes in blood gases stimulate the respiratory center. The first breath needs to be strong and deep to inflate the lungs.
  — The special features of fetal circulation cease to function after birth and degenerate or change into their postnatal state at birth or soon after.

- Discuss the hormonal and neural control of lactation.
  — Lactation refers to the production of milk by the mammary glands. For the first 2 or 3 days, the mammary glands secrete colostrum. After this, the glands produce milk.
  — The baby's suckling at the nipple sends signals to the hypothalamus; oxytocin is released; and this ejects milk from the mammary glands.
  — In response to the baby's suckling, the hypothalamus also releases prolactin-releasing hormone. This creates a surge in prolactin, which stimulates milk production for the next feeding period.

Postnatal Development

- Name and define six periods in postnatal development.
  — Neonatal period begins at the moment of birth and lasts until the end of the first four weeks.
  — Infancy lasts from the end of the first month to the end of the first year.
  — Childhood lasts from the end of the first year until puberty.
  — Adolescence begins at puberty and lasts until adulthood.
  — Adulthood is the period from adolescence to old age.
  — Senescence is the period of old age and ends in death.

LEARNING EXERCISES

Fertilization

1. Write the terms that match the following phrases about fertilization.

_____	Single cell that is product of fertilization
_____	Cells that surround ovulated secondary oocyte
_____	Process that weakens acrosomal membrane
_____	Length of time ovulated oocytes are fertile
_____	Usual site of fertilization

Preembryonic Period

1. Write the terms that match the following phrases about the preembryonic period.

_____ Developments during preembryonic period (3)

_____

_____

_____ Early cell divisions of the zygote

_____ Cells that are the result of cleavage

_____ Solid ball of cells resulting from cell division

_____ Hollow sphere of cells formed by fifth day

_____ Cluster of cells that becomes embryo

_____ Cavity within hollow sphere of cells

_____ Flattened cells around cavity of blastocyst

_____ Blastocyst cells that contribute to placenta

_____ Layer of uterine wall where implantation occurs

_____ Hormone secreted by the blastocyst

_____ Hormone that maintains the uterine lining

_____ Cluster of cells that forms primary germ layers

_____ Primary germ layers (3)

_____

_____

Embryonic Development

1. Complete the following statements by writing the correct words in the blanks.

The period of embryonic development lasts from the beginning of the _____ week after conception to the end of the _____ week. Three significant developments during this period are the formation of the _____ membranes, formation of the _____, and formation of all the body _____ systems. During this period the developing offspring is called an _____.

2. Match each of the following descriptive phrases with the correct extraembryonic membrane from the list.

_____ Forms a sac around the developing embryo

_____ Produces the primordial germ cells

_____ Becomes part of the umbilical cord

_____ Develops from the trophoblast

_____ Cushions and protects developing offspring

_____ Contributes to the formation of the placenta

_____ Develops fingerlike projections called villi

_____ Filled with fluid

A. amnion

B. allantois

C. chorion

D. yolk sac

3. Complete the following paragraph about the placenta by filling in the correct terms.

1. _____

2. _____

3. _____

4. _____

5. _____

6. _____

7. _____

8. _____

9. _____

The placenta develops as $\underline{1}$ from the embryo penetrate the $\underline{2}$ of the uterus. The $\underline{3}$ become highly vascular and extend to the $\underline{4}$ arteries and veins. The spaces in the endometrium are filled with maternal $\underline{5}$. This interface allows $\underline{6}$ and nutrients to diffuse from the mother's blood into the fetal blood. Metabolic wastes and $\underline{7}$ diffuse from the $\underline{8}$ into the $\underline{9}$.

4. Match each of the following tissues with the primary germ layer from which it is derived.

_____ Epithelial lining of the digestive tract

_____ Epidermis of the skin

_____ Cardiac muscle

_____ Nervous tissue

_____ Cartilage

_____ Hair, nails, glands of the skin

_____ Respiratory epithelium

_____ Epithelium lining the blood vessels

_____ Lining of the oral cavity

_____ Bone

_____ Dermis of the skin

_____ Epithelial lining of the vagina

A. ectoderm

B. mesoderm

C. endoderm

Fetal Development

1. Write the terms that match the following phrases about fetal development.

_____ First recognizable movements of fetus

_____ Protective coating over fetal skin

_____ Fine hair that covers fetal body

_____ Opening between the atria in the fetus

_____ Transports blood from placenta to fetus

_____ Allows blood to bypass fetal liver

Parturition and Lactation

1. Write the terms that match the following phrases about labor and delivery.

_____ Process of giving birth to an infant

_____ Series of contractions to expel fetus

_____ Hormone that inhibits uterine contractions

_____ Sensitizes uterus to effects of oxytocin

_____ Secretes oxytocin

_____ Act with oxytocin to stimulate contractions

_____ Type of feedback between oxytocin and uterus

_____ Longest stage of labor

_____ Stage of labor in which fetus is delivered

_____ Stage characterized by rhythmic contractions

_____ Final stage of labor

_____ Normal position, or presentation, of baby

2. Complete the following paragraph about the changes that take place in the lungs immediately after birth.

1. _____

2. _____

3. _____

4. _____

5. _____

6. _____

The fetal lungs are $\underline{1}$ and nonfunctional. When the $\underline{2}$ is cut, the oxygen supply from the mother ceases. Increasing $\underline{3}$ levels, decreasing $\underline{4}$, and $\underline{5}$ oxygen stimulate the respiratory center in the $\underline{6}$. The respiratory muscles contract and the baby takes its first breath. Usually this is strong and deep and inflates the alveoli.

3. Write the terms that match the following phrases about lactation.

_____ Refers to production and ejection of milk

_____ Hormone that stimulates milk production

_____ Hormone that stimulates milk ejection

_____ Inhibit milk production during pregnancy (2)

_____

_____ Yellowish fluid secreted before milk begins

4. Complete the following paragraph about the stimulation for milk production.

1. _____

2. _____

3. _____

4. _____

5. _____

6. _____

Each time a mother nurses her infant, impulses from the nipple to the <u>1</u> stimulate the release of <u>2</u>. This causes a temporary increase in <u>3</u>, which stimulates <u>4</u> for the next nursing period. If a mother stops nursing her baby, milk production <u>5</u> within a few <u>6</u>.

Postnatal Development

1. Identify the period of postnatal development described by each of the following.

_____ Lasts for about a month after birth

_____ Period of old age

_____ Lasts from the end of first year until puberty

_____ Lasts from end of first month to end of first year

_____ Puberty until adulthood

_____ Body weight generally triples

_____ Bladder and bowel controls are established

_____ Degenerative changes become significant

REVIEW QUESTIONS

1. What is the time period for prenatal development and postnatal development?

2. Why is capacitation necessary for fertilization?

3. Where does fertilization usually take place, and on what day of the menstrual cycle is it likely to occur?

4. What is the name of the single cell that is the result of fertilization? How many chromosomes does it have?

5. How long does the preembryonic period last, and what developmental events occur during this time?

6. What are the three parts of a blastocyst?

7. What hormone is secreted by the trophoblast cells, and what is its function?

8. Name the primary germ layers and list five derivatives from each one.

9. How long does the period of embryonic development last, and what takes place during this time?

10. What is the function of the (a) amnion; (b) chorion; (c) yolk sac; (d) allantois; (e) placenta?

11. How long does the fetal period development last, and what two fundamental processes take place during this period?

12. What is the purpose of each of the following: (a) umbilical arteries; (b) umbilical vein; (c) ductus venosus; (d) foramen ovale; (e) ductus arteriosus?

13. What is the normal length of time from fertilization until parturition?

14. What hormone from the posterior pituitary stimulates uterine contractions during labor?

15. List the three stages of labor and describe what takes place in each stage.

16. Why does a baby's first breath need to be especially strong and forceful?

17. What normally happens to each of the following after birth: (a) umbilical arteries; (b) umbilical vein; (c) ductus venosus; (d) foramen ovale; (e) ductus arteriosus?

18. When is colostrum produced? What is the difference between colostrum and milk?

19. What is the role of the mother's hypothalamus in providing milk for a nursing infant?

20. What effects do estrogen and progesterone have on the structure of the mammary glands?

21. How does the posterior pituitary affect the mammary glands?

22. Define six periods of life between birth and death.

CHAPTER QUIZ

1. Define the following terms:

   Capacitation

   Zygote

   Cleavage

   Chorionic villi

   Senescence

2. Arrange the following events in the correct sequence: (1) formation of the inner cell mass; (2) cleavage; (3) appearance of lanugo hair; (4) formation of the primary germ layers; (5) heart starts beating.
   (a) 1, 2, 4, 3, 5
   (b) 1, 2, 5, 3, 4
   (c) 4, 1, 2, 5, 3
   (d) 2, 1, 4, 5, 3
   (e) 2, 1, 4, 3, 5

3. Name the primary germ layer from which each of the following is derived.

   _____ Lens of the eye

   _____ Dermis of the skin

   _____ Lining of the digestive tract

   _____ Cartilage and bone

   _____ Epidermis of the skin

4. Name the extraembryonic membrane that does each of the following.

   _____ Functions in the formation of the placenta

   _____ Contributes to the development of umbilical vessels

   _____ Source of primordial germ cells

   _____ Provides a sac of fluid that allows freedom of movement

   _____ Produces blood for the embryo

5. The vessel between the umbilical vein and the inferior vena cava is the (a) umbilical artery; (b) ductus venosus; (c) ductus arteriosus; (d) internal iliac artery.

6. If a woman is 45 days past the beginning of her last menstrual period, the developing offspring is (a) in the cleavage stage of development; (b) in the preembryonic stage of development; (c) in the embryonic stage of development; (d) in the fetal stage of development; (e) in the implantation stage of development.

7. Which of the following is *not* true about the placenta? (a) it forms from both embryonic and maternal tissue; (b) blood-filled lacunae in the endometrium surround chorionic villi; (c) maternal blood enters the chorionic villi to provide oxygen for the fetus; (d) it is expelled in the placental stage of labor.

8. The birth of an infant is called (a) gestation; (b) parturition; (c) labor; (d) lactation.

9. Which of the following hormones is most responsible for continued milk production when breastfeeding an infant? (a) human chorionic gonadotropin; (b) placental lactogen; (c) estrogen; (d) prolactin; (e) oxytocin.

10. Which of the following does *not* refer to the neonatal period? (a) begins at the moment of birth; (b) temperature-regulating mechanisms may not be fully developed; (c) baby learns to smile and laugh; (d) foramen ovale normally closes.

USING CLINICAL KNOWLEDGE

1. Match the definitions on the left with the correct term from the column on the right by placing the corresponding letter in the space before the definition. Not all terms will be used.

_____ Act of giving birth to an infant	A. Amnion
_____ Innermost fetal membrane	B. Eclampsia
_____ Preparations that reduce or inhibit uterine contractions	C. Embryo
	D. Eutocia
_____ Woman who has borne more than one child	E. Fetus
_____ An agent that causes physical defects in a developing embryo	F. Lochia
	G. Multipara
_____ Period during which organ systems develop	H. Neonate
_____ Synthetic oxytocin	I. Parturition
_____ Good, normal childbirth	J. Pitocin
_____ Vaginal discharge during the first two weeks after childbirth	K. Teratogen
	L. Tocolytics
_____ Infant during first month after birth	

2. Write the meaning of the following abbreviations.

_____ GYN

_____ HCG

_____ SIDS

_____ EDD

_____ FHR

3. Spelling is important in scientific and medical applications because only one or two incorrect letters may change the meaning. Circle the correctly spelled word for each of the following pairs.

gestation	jestation
corion	chorion
senescence	senesance
zona pellucida	zona pelucida
clostrum	colostrum

4. Write the meaning of the underlined portion of each word on the line preceding the word.

_____ <u>amnio</u>rrhea

_____ <u>contra</u>ceptive

_____ pseudocyesis

_____ primigravida

_____ nullipara

_____ prenatal

5. Use your knowledge of word parts from all chapters to write definitions of the words in question #4.

amniorrhea _____

_____

contraceptive _____

_____

pseudocyesis _____

_____

primigravida _____

_____

nullipara _____

_____

prenatal _____

_____

6. There were complications in Clacy's pregnancy because of an abnormal implantation of the placenta in the lower portion of the uterus.

(a) What is the clinical term for this condition?

(b) During which prenatal period does the placenta develop?

(c) Name three hormones produced by the placenta.

FUN AND GAMES

Each of the answers in this puzzle is a term from this chapter on development. Fill in the answers to the clues by using syllables from the list that is provided. The number of syllables in each word is indicated by the number in parentheses after the clue. The number of letters in each word is indicated by the number of spaces provided. All syllables in the list are to be used and no syllable is used more than once unless it is duplicated in the list.

A	CO	IN	NIX	OR	TOC
AD	E	LA	NU	OX	TROPH
AM	E	LA	O	PAR	TRUM
AT	E	LES	O	PLA	TU
BLAST	FOR	LOS	O	RI	U
CAS	GAN	MEN	O	SA	VAGE
CEN	GEN	MOR	O	SE	VAL
CENCE	GEN	NATE	O	SIS	VER
CENCE	GO	NE	O	TA	Y
CHOR	GOTE	NES	ON	TER	ZY
CLEA	I	NI	ON	TION	

Product of fertilization (2)   _ _ _ _ _ _

Early mitotic cell divisions after fertilization (2)   _ _ _ _ _ _ _

Solid ball of blastomeres (3)   _ _ _ _ _ _

Cells around the blastocele (3)   _ _ _ _ _ _ _ _ _

Membrane around embryo/fetus (3)   _ _ _ _ _ _ _

Extraembryonic membrane that contributes to placenta (3)   _ _ _ _ _ _ _

Site of nutrient and gaseous exchange for fetus (3)   _ _ _ _ _ _ _ _

Formation of body organs (6)   _ _ _ _ _ _ _ _ _ _ _

Fine hair that covers fetus (3)   _ _ _ _ _ _

Mixture of sebum and cells on fetal skin (6)   _ _ _ _ _ _ _ _ _ _ _

Birth of an infant (4)   _ _ _ _ _ _ _ _ _

Opening between R & L atria in fetus (6)   _ _ _ _ _ _ _ _ _ _ _ _ _

Hormone that stimulates milk ejection (4)   _ _ _ _ _ _ _ _

Secreted before milk production begins (3)   _ _ _ _ _ _ _ _

Infant during first four weeks after birth (3)   _ _ _ _ _ _ _

Period from puberty to adulthood (4)   _ _ _ _ _ _ _ _ _ _

Period of old age (3)   _ _ _ _ _ _ _ _

Substance that causes physical defects in embryo (4)   _ _ _ _ _ _ _ _

Answers to Learning Exercises

CHAPTER 1

Anatomy and Physiology
1. Anatomy
2. Physiology
3. Function, structure
4. Surface anatomy
   Cytology
   Embryology
   Immunology
   Pharmacology
   Pathology

Levels of Organization
1. Chemical, cellular, tissues, organs, body systems, total organism
2. Cell
3. Tissue

Organ Systems
1. Integumentary
2. Skeletal
3. Digestive
4. Respiratory
5. Urinary
6. Endocrine
7. Lymphatic
8. Nervous
9. Cardiovascular
10. Lymphatic
11. Digestive
12. Nervous
13. Endocrine
14. Cardiovascular
15. Urinary
16. Muscular
17. Lymphatic
18. Integumentary
19. Skeletal
20. Reproductive

Life Processes
1. (Any order) Organization, metabolism, responsiveness, movement, reproduction, growth, differentiation, respiration, digestion, excretion
2. Catabolism

3. Anabolism is a building up process in which complex substances are synthesized from simpler ones.
4. (Any order) Water, oxygen, nutrients, heat, pressure

Homeostasis
1. Homeostasis
2. Stressor
3. Negative feedback
4. Positive feedback

Anatomical Terms
1. Body is **erect**.
   Face is **forward**.
   Arms are **at sides**.
   Palms are **forward**.
   Feet and toes are **directed forward**.
2. Superior
   Proximal
   Deep
   Anterior to
   Visceral
3. Midsagittal (median sagittal)
   Transverse (horizontal)
   Frontal (coronal)
   Sagittal
4. Dorsal cavity
   Ventral cavity
   Cranial cavity
   Thoracic cavity
   Abdominal cavity
   Spinal cavity
   Pelvic cavity
5. A. Right hypochondriac
   B. Umbilical
   C. Left iliac (inguinal)
   D. Epigastric
   E. Left lumbar
   F. Left hypochondriac
   G. Right lumbar
   H. Hypogastric
   I. Right iliac (inguinal)
6. A. Otic
   B. Sternal
   C. Brachial

D. Antebrachial
E. Leg (crural)
F. Oral
G. Pectoral (mammary)
H. Umbilical (navel)
I. Inguinal
J. Femoral
K. Occipital
L. Sacral
M. Carpal
N. Popliteal
O. Pedal
P. Cervical
Q. Axillary
R. Lumbar
S. Gluteal
T. Palmar

Concepts of Terminology
1. (1) prefix
   (2) root
   (3) suffix
2. Gastr- is the root and it means stomach
3. root: skelet; means a dried, hard body
   suffix: -al; means pertaining to

CHAPTER 2

Elements
1. Matter is defined as anything that takes up space and has mass.
2. An element is defined as the simplest form of matter; it cannot be broken into a simpler form by ordinary chemical means.
3. H = Hydrogen; Mg = Magnesium; C = Carbon; O = Oxygen; K = Potassium; P = Phosphorus
4. Sodium = Na; Nitrogen = N; Calcium = Ca; Iron = Fe; Chlorine = Cl; Sulfur = S

Structure of Atoms

1.

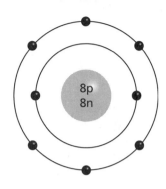

2. Particle: neutron, electron, proton
   Location: nucleus, orbitals, nucleus
   Charge: 0, −, +
   Mass: 1, negligible, 1
3. 19 protons, 20 neutrons, 19 electrons
4. 8 electrons
5. Isotopes; neutrons
6. Radioactive isotopes

Chemical Bonds

1. C, D, E, A, B, C

Compounds and Molecules

1. Atom
   Molecule
   Compound
   Molecule
2. Calcium, 1 atom
   Carbon, 1 atom
   Oxygen, 3 atoms

Chemical Reactions

1. Equation: $H_2CO_3 \rightarrow H_2O + CO_2$
   Type of reaction: Decomposition
   Reactants: H_2CO_3
   Products: H_2O and CO_2
   Equation: $N_2 + 3H_2 \rightarrow 2NH_3$
   Type of reaction: Composition, Synthesis
   Reactants: N_2 and H_2
   Products: NH_3, ammonia
   Equation: $MgCl_2 + 2NaOH \rightarrow Mg(OH)_2 + 2NaCl$
   Type of reaction: Double replacement
   Reactants: $MgCl_2$ and $NaOH$
   Products: $Mg(OH)_2$ and $NaCl$
   Equation: $C_7H_6O_3 + C_2H_4O_2 \rightarrow C_9H_8O_4 + H_2O$

   Type of reaction: Composition, Synthesis
   Reactants: $C_7H_6O_3$ and $C_2H_4O_2$
   Products: $C_9H_8O_4$ and H_2O
2. Exergonic, endergonic
3. I (Grind up the reactants)
   I (Add a catalyst)
   I (Use more concentrated solutions)
   D (Dilute one reactant)
   D (Cool the reaction mixture)
   I (Increase the temperature)
4. The reaction is reversible. It may proceed in either direction.

Mixtures, Solutions, and Suspension

1. (c) solvent
2. (a) are clear
3. Mixture (sugar and salt)
   Suspension (blood cells and plasma)
   Solution (sugar and water)
   Suspension (cytoplasm of the cell)
   Mixture (sand and water)

Acids, Bases, and Buffers

1. Electrolytes
2. Base (accepts hydrogen ions)
   Acid (reacts with a buffer to form weak acid)
   Acid (has sour taste)
   Acid (reacts with OH ions to form water)
   Acid (has pH of 3.5)
   Base (has slippery, soapy feeling)
   Acid (donates protons)
   Base (has pH of 8.7)
3. $HC_2H_3O_2$ reacts; H_2O is formed
   $NaC_2H_3O_2$ reacts; $NaCl$ is formed

Organic Compounds

1. Carbon, hydrogen, oxygen
2. Glucose, fructose, and galactose
3. Disaccharide
4. Complex polysaccharides
5. Nitrogen
   Amino acids
   Essential
6. Glycerol and fatty acids
   Saturated
   Phospholipids
7. DNA

RNA
Nucleotides
Deoxyribose
DNA
C, H, O, N, P
RNA
ATP
8. A (glucose)
   A (glycogen)
   C (amino acids)
   C (hemoglobin)
   B (steroids)
   D (RNA)
   D (nucleotides)
   A (disaccharides)
   B (glycerol)
   B (triglycerides)

CHAPTER 3

Structure of the Generalized Cell

1. Structural support, channels for passage of materials, receptor sites, carrier molecules, identification markers for immunity.
2. G (cell membrane)
   F (centriole)
   E (chromatin)
   L (cilia)
   I (Golgi apparatus)
   H (mitochondria)
   J (nuclear pore)
   D (nucleolus)
   C (nucleus)
   A (ribosome)
   K (RER)
   B (SER)
3. Mitochondria
   Lysosome
   Golgi apparatus
   Ribosomes
   Centrioles
   Cilia
   Endoplasmic reticulum
   Chromatin
   Flagella
   Nucleolus
   Cytoplasm
   Cell membrane
   Nucleus
   Microfilaments
   Microtubules

Cell Functions

1. Osmosis

Simple diffusion
Facilitated diffusion
2. Active transport
Endocytosis
Passive transport
Exocytosis
Active transport
Passive transport
Endocytosis
3. A is hypertonic.
A will increase in volume.
4. Anaphase, Prophase, Metaphase
5. Mitosis: Somatic, 2, 46
Meiosis: Gametes, 4, 23
6. Mitosis (cell division)
7. mRNA: AUG/UGU/UAC/AUU/
CAA/AAC
tRNA: UAC/ACA/AUG/UAA/GUU/
UUG

CHAPTER 4

Body Tissues

1. A tissue is a group of similar cells collected together by an intercellular matrix.
2. Histology
3. Epithelial, connective, muscular, nervous
4. Epithelial tissues consist of closely packed cells with very little intercellular matrix. They have one free surface, have no blood (vascular) supply, and reproduce quickly. These tissues cover the body, line body cavities, and cover the organs within the body cavities. The cells may be flat (squamous), cuboidal, or columnar in shape.
5. Simple cuboidal
Kidneys
Stratified squamous
Skin
Pseudostratified ciliated columnar
Respiratory passages
6. Endocrine
Exocrine
Exocrine
Exocrine
Endocrine
7. B
D
G

E
F
8. Collagenous (white)
Macrophage
Areolar (loose connective tissue)
Adipose
Dense fibrous
Perichondrium
Fibrocartilage
Bone
Haversian system (osteon)
Osteocytes
Blood (vascular)
Erythrocytes
9. Areolar (loose)
White collagenous (A)
Yellow elastic (B)
10. Hyaline cartilage
Chondrin (A)
Chondrocyte (B)
Lacuna (C)
11. Bone or osseous connective tissue
Lamellae (A)
Haversian (osteonic) canal (B)
Canaliculi (C)
12. Skeletal
Sarcolemma (A)
Actin and myosin
13. Smooth (visceral)
Blood vessels and wall of hollow body organs
14. Cardiac
Intercalated disc (B)
Heart
15. Neurons
Dendrites
Axons
Neuroglia

Inflammation and Tissue Repair

1. (a) redness, heat
(b) pain, swelling
2. F (scar tissue)
R (surface abrasions)
R (cells identical)
F (granulation tissue)
R (tissues capable of mitosis)
F (skeletal muscle)
F (collagen fibers)

Body Membranes

1. Connective tissue membranes
Mucous membranes
Mucous membrane
Serous membrane

Parietal
Visceral
Pleura
Pericardium
Peritoneum
Synovial
Meninges
Dura mater
Arachnoid
Pia mater

CHAPTER 5

Structure of the Skin

1. Skin, hair, nails, and glands
2. Hypodermis
Stratum basale
Stratum basale
Stratum germinativum
Dermis
Stratum spinosum
Hypodermis
Stratum lucidum
Stratum granulosum
Stratum corneum
Dermis
Dermis
Hypodermis
Stratum basale
Dermis
3. C (arrector pili muscle)
H (blood vessel)
A (epidermis)
G (hair bulb)
F (sebaceous gland)
B (stratum basale)
E (stratum corneum)
D (sweat gland)

Skin Color

1. Melanin
2. Carotene
3. Blood vessels in the dermis
4. As cells with increased melanin are pushed to the surface, die, and are sloughed off, the tan lightens because the new cells do not have as much melanin.

Epidermal Derivatives

1. Follicle
Arrector pili
Stratum basale
Medulla
Lunula
Sebaceous
Ceruminous
Merocrine

Sudoriferous
Bulb
Eponychium
Apocrine

Functions of the Skin

1. (a) protection, (b) sensory reception, (c) regulation of body temperature, (d) synthesis of vitamin D
2. Keratin
3. Oily secretions of sebaceous glands
4. Melanin
5. Dermis
6. (a) Blood vessels dilate to bring more blood to the surface to radiate heat from the body. In cold, they constrict to conserve heat inside the body. (b) In heat, sweat glands actively produce perspiration which carries large quantities of heat to the surface. Evaporation then cools the body. In cold, sweat glands are inactive.
7. Precursors for vitamin D are in the skin and when exposed to ultraviolet from the sun, vitamin D is formed.

Burns

1. 3 (requires skin grafts)
   2, 3 (stratum basale damaged)
   1 (heals by regeneration)
   1, 2 (becomes red)
   3 (involves subcutaneous tissue)
   1, 2 (painful)
   2 (blisters)
   1 (superficial)
   2 (may produce scarring)
   2, 3 (involves the dermis)
   3 (severe scarring)
   3 (nerve endings destroyed)
2. (a) 27%
   (b) infection and fluid loss

CHAPTER 6

Overview of Skeletal System

1. (a) support, (b) protection, (c) movement, (d) storage, (e) blood cell formation.
2. C   (closely packed osteons)
   S   (contains red bone marrow)
   S   (trabeculae)
   C   (canaliculi radiate from lacunae)
   S   (contains irregular spaces)
3. F   (has diploe of spongy bone)
   L   (vertical dimension longer than horizontal)
   S   (roughly cube shaped)
   S   (primarily spongy bone)
   S   (bones in wrist and ankle)
   L   (bones in thigh and arm)
   F   (spongy bone between two compact layers)
4. Diaphysis
   Epiphysis
   Periosteum
   Medullary cavity
   Articular cartilage
   Endosteum
5. Condyle
   Foramen
   Fossa
   Sinus
   Facet
   Trochanter
6. Osteogenesis/ossification
   Osteoblasts
   Osteocytes
   Osteoclasts
   Intramembranous
   Endochondral
   Epiphyseal plate
   Osteoblasts
   Osteoclasts
   Endochondral
7. 206 (complete skeleton)
   80 (axial skeleton)
   126 (appendicular skeleton)

Axial Skeleton

1. Frontal (1), parietal (2), occipital (1), temporal (2), ethmoid (1), sphenoid (1).
2. Nasal (2), maxillae (2), zygomatic (2), inferior nasal conchae (2), lacrimal (2), palatine (2), mandible (1), vomer (1).
3. Occipital (foramen magnum)
   Temporal (auditory meatus)
   Frontal (supraorbital foramen)
   Temporal (mastoid process)
   Sphenoid (optic foramen)
   Ethmoid (cribriform plate)
   Sphenoid (sella turcica)
   Mandible (ramus)
4. Hyoid
5. Atlas (first cervical vertebra)

Thoracic (articulate with ribs)
Body/centrum (weight bearing portion)
Manubrium (superior portion of breastbone)
Axis (second cervical vertebra)
Cervical (type of vertebrae in neck)
Lumbar (heavy bodies and blunt processes)
Sternum (another name for breastbone)
Intervertebral discs (cartilaginous pads)

6. 7 pr=14 (true ribs)
   7 (cervical vertebrae)
   5 pr=10 (false ribs)
   12 (thoracic vertebrae)
   5 (lumbar vertebrae)
   7 pr=14 (vertebrosternal ribs)
   2 pr=4 (vertebral ribs)
   3 pr=6 (vertebrochondral ribs)
7. R   (mandible)
   L   (frontal)
   D   (temporal)
   N   (nasal)
   Q   (maxilla)
   E   (occipital)
   P   (zygomatic)
   M   (sphenoid)
   O   (lacrimal)
   A   (parietal)
   J   (ramus)
   K   (coronal suture)
   G   (mastoid process)
   I   (mandibular condyle)
   H   (styloid process)
   F   (auditory meatus)
   B   (squamosal suture)
   C   (lambdoidal suture)

Appendicular Skeleton

1. Clavicle (anterior bone of pectoral girdle)
   Scapula (posterior bone of pectoral girdle)
   Scapula (has acromion and spine)
   Humerus (large bone in arm)
   Radius (bone on lateral side of forearm)
   Ulna (bone on medial side of forearm)
   Carpals (wrist bones)
   Metacarpals (form palm of the hand)

Phalanges (form fingers and toes)
Ulna (articulates with trochlea of humerus)
Radius (articulates with capitulum)
Olecranon process (projection on ulna)

2. Ilium
Ischium
Pubis
Acetabulum
Condyles
Tibia
Fibula
Calcaneus
Talus
Patella
Sacrum
Femur

3. Male pelvis:
Arch less than 90°
Inlet narrow, heart-shaped
Cavity narrow, deep, funnel-shaped
Female pelvis:
Arch more than 90°
Inlet wider and oval
Cavity broad, oval, shallow

4. The portion of the pelvis between the flared wings of the ilium bones is called the **false** pelvis. The portion inferior to the pelvic brim is the **true** pelvis.

5. A   Frontal
B   Humerus
C   Os coxa (ilium)
D   Carpals
E   Femur
F   Patella
G   Metatarsals
H   Mandible
I   Clavicle
J   Sternum
K   Radius
L   Phalanges
M   Tibia
N   Phalanges

6. A   Parietal
B   Scapula
C   Humerus
D   Ulna
E   Sacrum
F   Metacarpals
G   Fibula

H   Talus
I   Tarsals
J   Occipital
K   Cervical vertebrae
L   Ribs
M   Lumbar vertebrae
N   Radius
O   Femur
P   Tibia
Q   Calcaneus

Fractures and Fracture Repair

1. open
comminuted
transverse
displaced
spiral

2. (a) closed
(b) incomplete
(c) 4 (Bony callus)
   1 (Fracture hematoma)
   5 (Remodeling)
   2 (Procallus)
   3 (Fibrocartilaginous callus)

Articulations

1. Synarthrosis (sutures)
Amphiarthrosis (slightly movable)
Diarthrosis (meniscus)
Synarthrosis (immovable)
Diarthrosis (elbow and knee)
Diarthrosis (ball and socket)
Amphiarthrosis (ribs to sternum)
Diarthrosis (may have bursae)
Diarthrosis (joint capsule)
Amphiarthrosis (symphysis pubis)

CHAPTER 7

Characteristics and Functions of the Muscular System

1. C (striated and involuntary)
B (spindle shaped fibers)
A (multinucleated and cylindrical)
B (found in blood vessels)
C (found in the heart)

2. Excitability, contractility, extensibility, elasticity

a. Movement, posture, heat production

Structure of Skeletal Muscle

1. Insertion

Endomysium
Myosin
Fasciculus
Origin
Aponeurosis
Sarcolemma
Actin
Sarcomere
Thin/actin

2. Muscle fibers must be stimulated before they can contract, therefore they have an abundant **nerve supply**. The blood supply delivers **oxygen** and **nutrients** for contraction.

Contraction of Skeletal Muscle

1. 7   Energized myosin
2   Acetylcholine is released
8   Power stroke pulls
6   Calcium reacts
3   Acetylcholine reacts
1   Nerve impulse
5   Calcium ions are released
4   Impulse travels

2. Threshold (liminal)
All-or-none
Subthreshold (subliminal)
Motor unit
Summation
Tetany
Treppe
Tone
Isotonic
Isometric

3. ATP
Creatine phosphate
Myoglobin
Lactic acid
$CO_2 + H_2O$ + energy (ATP)

4. The muscle that has a primary role in providing a movement is called the **prime mover**. Muscles that assist this muscle are called **synergists** and muscles that oppose the movement are called **antagonists**.

5. E   (extension of foot to stand on tiptoes)
G   (movement of arm toward the midline)
B   (straightening the arm at the elbow)
I   (turning the palm of the hand forward)
H   (turning the head from side to side)

A (moving elbow to put hand on shoulder)
L (turning the sole of foot inward)
F (spreading the fingers apart)
C (tilting head backward)
K (drawing circles on chalkboard)

Skeletal Muscle Groups
1. Action (adductor)
   Direction of fibers (rectus)
   Size (maximus)
   Location (gluteus)
   Shape (deltoid)
   Number of origins (biceps)
   Origin/insertion (brachioradialis)
   Location (pectoralis)
2. Frontalis
   Orbicularis oris
   Temporalis
   Masseter
   Orbicularis oculi
   Sternocleidomastoid
   Diaphragm
   Pectoralis major
   Latissimus dorsi
   Deltoid
   Triceps brachii
   Biceps brachii
   Brachialis
   Iliopsoas
   Tensor fasciae latae
   Gluteus maximus
   Adductors
   Quadriceps femoris
   Biceps femoris
   Semimembranosus
   Semitendinosus
   Gastrocnemius
   Soleus (also peroneus)
   Tibialis anterior
3. A Frontalis
   B Orbicularis oculi
   C Orbicularis oris
   D Temporalis
   E Zygomaticus
   F Buccinator
   G Trapezius
   H Infraspinatus
   I Latissimus dorsi
   J Gluteus maximus
   K Sternocleidomastoid
   L Deltoid
   M Triceps brachii

N Gluteus medius
4. A Iliopsoas
   B Adductor longus
   C Gracilis
   D Vastus medialis
   E Tensor fasciae latae
   F Sartorius
   G Rectus femoris
   H Vastus lateralis
   I Gluteus medius
   J Vastus lateralis
   K Semitendinosus
   L Biceps femoris
   M Gluteus maximus
   N Gracilis
   O Semimembranosus
   P Gastrocnemius

CHAPTER 8

Functions of the Nervous System
1. The activities of the nervous system are grouped into three functional categories. These are **sensory, integrative, and motor**.

Organization of the Nervous System
1. The two components of the central nervous system are the **brain** and **spinal cord**.
2. The two divisions of the peripheral nervous system are the **afferent**, or sensory division, and the **efferent**, or motor, division.
3. The autonomic nervous system is a part of the **efferent (motor)** division of the peripheral nervous system.

Nerve Tissue
1. Dendrite
   Myelin
   Afferent (sensory)
   Node of Ranvier
   Interneurons (association neurons)
   Axon
   Neurilemma
2. A Nucleus
   B Dendrite
   C Schwann cell (neurilemma)
   D Axon collateral
   E Myelin

F Cell body
G Node of Ranvier
H Axon cylinder
I Telodendria
3. Astrocyte
   Microglia
   Oligodendroglia
   Schwann cell
   Ependyma
   Satellite cell

Nerve Impulses
1. Two functional characteristics of neurons are **irritability (excitability)** and **conductivity**.
2. At rest, the outside of a neuron is **positive** (charge) and has a higher concentration of **sodium** ions relative to the inside. A stimulus changes the permeability of the membrane and it depolarizes. During depolarization, **sodium** ions diffuse into the cell. This creates an **action** potential, or nerve impulse. During repolarization, **potassium** ions diffuse out of the cell. At the conclusion of the **stimulus**, the **sodium/potassium** pump restores the ionic conditions of a resting membrane. The minimum stimulus required to initiate a nerve impulse is called a **threshold (liminal)** stimulus.
3. 11, 9, 6, 3, 13, 7, 4, 1, 12, 8, 5, 2, 10
4. H (rapid conduction)
   I (region of communication)
   E (diffuses across synaptic cleft)
   G (time during which a neuron…)
   C (synaptic transmission…)
   F (functional unit of nervous system)
   B (single neuron synapses…)
   D (synaptic transmission …)
   A (several neurons synapse…)

Central Nervous System
1. 4 (arachnoid)
   1 (epidural)
   5 (subarachnoid)

2 (dura mater)
6 (pia mater)
3 (subdural)
2. A Parietal lobe
   B Occipital lobe
   C Cerebellum
   D Medulla oblongata
   E Corpus callosum
   F Frontal lobe
   G Midbrain
   H Pons
3. Cerebellum
   Brain stem
   Diencephalon
   Medulla oblongata
   Hypothalamus
   Pons
   Midbrain
   Cerebellum
   Medulla oblongata
   Pons
4. 7, 2, 6, 9, 4, 1, 3, 8, 5
5. A (central canal)
   D (dorsal horn)
   B (column of white matter)
   F (spinal nerve)
   E (dorsal root ganglion)
   C (ventral root)
6. The spinal cord consists of a central core of white matter surrounded by gray matter. The spinal cord consists of a central core of **gray** matter surrounded by **white** matter. Two enlargements of the spinal cord are in the thoracic and lumbar regions. Two enlargements of the spinal cord are in the **cervical** and **sacral** regions.
   The dorsal, lateral, and ventral horns contain bundles of nerve fibers, called nerve tracts. The dorsal, lateral, and ventral **columns** contain bundles of nerve fibers, called nerve tracts.
   Ascending tracts carry motor impulses to the brain. Ascending tracts carry **sensory** impulses to the brain.
   Corticospinal tracts are ascending tracts that begin in the cerebral cortex. Corticospinal tracts are **descending** tracts that begin in the cerebral cortex.

Peripheral Nervous System
1. Within a nerve, each individual nerve fiber has a connective tissue covering called **endoneurium**. The nerve itself is covered by connective tissue called **epineurium**.
2. Three nerves that are sensory only: Olfactory, optic, vestibulocochlear
   Nerve to the muscles of facial expression: Facial
   Three nerves that function in eye movement: Oculomotor, abducens, trochlear
   Nerve that is likely to be involved if you have a toothache in the lower jaw: Mandibular branch of the trigeminal nerve
   Nerve to the muscles of mastication: Trigeminal
   Nerve that allows you to nod your head: Spinal accessory
3. 31 pr (number of spinal nerves)
   Dorsal (spinal nerve root...)
   Plexus (complex network...)
   8 pr (number of cervical nerves)
   Ventral (spinal nerve...)
   Brachial (nerve plexus that supplies...)
   Cervical (nerve plexus that gives rise to the phrenic nerve)
   Lumbosacral (nerve plexus that gives rise to the sciatic nerve)
4. Single arrow red; two arrows blue
   Preganglionic is CNS to ganglion
   Postganglionic is ganglion to effector
   Autonomic effector has asterisk
5. *Checks (√) for Sympathetic*
   Arises from thoracic and lumbar regions
   Has short preganglionic fibers
   Also called "fight-or-flight"
   Cholinergic preganglionic fibers
   Adrenergic postganglionic fibers
   Dilates pupils of the eyes
   Increases heart rate
   Dilates blood vessels to skeletal muscles
   Checks (√) for Parasympathetic
   Has terminal ganglia
   Also called the craniosacral division
   Cholinergic preganglionic fibers
   Also called "rest-and-repose" system
   Has short postganglionic fibers
   Cholinergic postganglionic fibers
   Increases digestive enzymes
   Constricts the bronchi

CHAPTER 9

Receptors and Sensations
1. Senses with receptors that are widely distributed within the body are called **general** senses. If the receptors are localized in a specific region, they are called **special** senses.
2. Photoreceptor
   Baroreceptor
   Thermoreceptor
   Nociceptor
   Chemoreceptor
3. Sensory adaptation occurs when certain receptors are continually stimulated and no longer respond unless the stimulus becomes more intense.

General Senses
1. Check (√) before each of the following:
   Pacinian corpuscles -mechanoreceptors
   Pain / nociceptors
   Mechanoreceptors / proprioception
2. **Thermoreceptors** exhibit rapid sensory adaptation. **Nociceptors** may send impulses after the stimulus is removed.

Gustatory Sense
1. Gustatory

Papillae
Taste hair cells
Chemoreceptors
2. Sweet, sour, salty, bitter
Facial nerve
Glossopharyngeal nerve
Parietal lobe

Olfactory Sense
1. Nasal cavity
2. I, temporal
3. taste, smell

Visual Sense
1. Lacrimal
Conjunctiva
Sclera
Cornea
Choroid
Pupil
Aqueous humor
Iris
Ciliary
Produce aqueous humor
Retina
Rods and cones
Blind spot (optic disk)
Fovea centralis
Vitreous humor
2. Refraction
3. Accommodation is the adjustment needed to focus light rays for **close** vision. To focus light rays from close objects, the ciliary muscle **contracts**, which **decreases** the tension on the suspensory ligaments. When this happens, the lens becomes **thicker** and light rays are bent **more**. In addition, the pupil **constricts**.
4. C (anterior cavity)
   H (choroid)
   F (ciliary body)
   D (cornea)
   A (eyelid)
   B (iris)
   K (lens)
   L (optic nerve)
   J (posterior cavity)
   I (retina)
   G (sclera)
   E (suspensory ligaments)
5. Cones
   Rhodopsin
   Cones
   Red, blue, green

Rods
Rhodopsin
Rods
Vitamin A
Optic disk
Rods
6. 3 (optic chiasma)
   2 (optic nerve)
   7 (occipital lobe)
   4 (optic tract)
   5 (thalamus)
   1 (photoreceptors)
   6 (optic radiations)

Auditory Sense
1. F (ampulla)
   E (auditory tube)
   J (auricle)
   D (cochlea)
   I (external auditory canal)
   G (incus)
   K (malleus)
   A (semicircular canals)
   L (stapes)
   H (tympanic membrane)
   B (vestibule)
   C (vestibulocochlear nerve)
2. Bony labyrinth
   Membranous labyrinth
   Endolymph
   Perilymph
   Cochlea
   Cochlear duct
   Basilar membrane
   Vestibular membrane
   Basilar membrane
3. 1. Tympanic membrane
   2. Malleus
   3. Incus
   4. Stapes
   5. Perilymph
   6. Endolymph
   7. Hair cells
   8. Tectorial membrane
   9. Basilar membrane
   10. Oscillation

Sense of Equilibrium
1. Dynamic equilibrium
   Static equilibrium
   Macula
   Utricle
   Saccule
   Otoliths
   Crista ampullaris
   Ampulla of semicircular canals

CHAPTER 10

Introduction to the Endocrine System
1. E (acts through hormones)
   N (effect is localized)
   N (acts through electrical impulses)
   N (effect is of short-term duration)
   E (effect is generalized and long-term)
2. Exocrine glands have **ducts** that carry the secretory product to a surface. In contrast, **endocrine glands** are ductless and secrete their product directly into the **blood** for transport to the target tissue.

Characteristics of Hormones
1. Protein
   Steroids
   Target cells
   Cell membrane
   Cytoplasm
   Neural
   Humoral (negative feedback)
   Hormonal
2. 1. Protein
   2. Adenyl cyclase
   3. Cyclic AMP
   4. ATP
   5. Hormone
   6. Cyclic AMP
   7. Steroid
   8. Receptor
   9. Nucleus
   10. DNA

Endocrine Glands and their Hormones
1. D (adrenal gland)
   E (ovaries)
   H (pancreas)
   B (parathyroid)
   A (pineal gland)
   F (pituitary gland)
   C (thymus)
   G (thyroid)
   I (testes)
2. B (secretes ADH)
   A (stimulated by releasing hormones)
   A (secretes prolactin)
   B (derived from nervous tissue)

B   (secretes oxytocin)
A   (derived from embryonic oral cavity)
A   (secretes TSH)
A   (secretes growth hormone)
A   (secretes ACTH)
B   (regulated by nerve stimulation)

3. Thyroid-stimulating hormone
Adrenocorticotropic hormone
Luteinizing hormone
Oxytocin
Antidiuretic hormone
Follicle-stimulating hormone
Growth hormone (somatotropin)
Oxytocin
Luteinizing hormone (ICSH)
Prolactin

4. C   (secreted by parafollicular cells)
T   (requires iodine for production)
P   (increases blood calcium levels)
T   (secreted by thyroid follicles)
T   (increases rate of metabolism)
C   (reduces blood calcium levels)
P   (increases osteoclast activity)
P   (hyposecretion leads to nerve excitability)

5. Medulla
Mineralocorticoids
Aldosterone
Cortex
Cortisol
Aldosterone
Cortisol
Gonadocorticoids
Epinephrine
Norepinephrine

6. Insulin
Glucagon
Glucagon
Insulin
Insulin
Glucagon
Glucagon
Insulin
Insulin

7. G   7   (testosterone)

C   10   (melatonin)
H   4   (thymosin)
B   5   (estrogen)
D   6   (HCG)
F   9   (gastrin)
E   1   (secretin)
B   8   (progesterone)
E   2   (cholecystokinin)
A   3   (atrial peptin)

Prostaglandins

1. Prostaglandins are similar to hormones but they are different in many ways. They are derivatives of **arachidonic acid** and the cells that produce them are **scattered (distributed)** throughout the body.

2. In contrast to hormones, the effects of prostaglandins are **localized, immediate**, and **short-term**.

CHAPTER 11

Functions and Characteristics of the Blood

1. 7.35 to 7. 45
5 liters
Gases
Nutrients
Waste products
Body temperature
Fluid and electrolyte balance
pH

Composition of the Blood

1. Blood is **55%** plasma and **45%** formed elements.

2. Albumin -Osmotic pressure.
36% -Lipid transport/immune reactions.
Fibrinogen -4%.

3. Nonprotein molecules: amino acids, urea, uric acid.
Nutrients: amino acids, glucose, fatty acids.
Gases: oxygen and carbon dioxide.
Electrolytes: Na^+, K^+, Ca^{++}, Cl^-, HCO_3^-, PO_4^{-3}.

4. Erythrocytes
Leukocytes
Thrombocytes

5. E   (basophil)
B   (eosinophil)
D   (erythrocyte)
F   (lymphocyte)

C   (monocyte)
A   (neutrophil)

6. Erythrocytes
Reticulocytes
4.5 to 6 million
Hemoglobin
Diapedesis
5000 to 9000
Neutrophil
Eosinophil
Basophil
Monocyte
Lymphocyte
Neutrophil
Monocyte
Neutrophil
Monocyte
Basophil
Eosinophil
Blood clotting
250,000 to 500,000
Megakaryocyte

7. Hemocytoblast
Erythropoietin
Iron
Vitamin B_{12}
Folic acid
Intrinsic factor
120 days or 4 months
Spleen
Liver
Bilirubin

Hemostasis

1. Vascular constriction
Platelet plug formation
Vitamin K
Calcium
Fibrinolysis

2. Substance A = Prothrombin activator
Substance B = Prothrombin
Substance C = Thrombin
Substance D = Fibrinogen

Blood Typing and Transfusion

1. A | A | anti-B | A and O | A and AB
B | B | anti-A | B and O | B and AB
AB | A and B | none | A, B, O, AB | AB
O | none | anti-A and anti-B | O | A, B, AB, O

2. Rh+ (D)
None
None

anti-Rh (anti-D)

3. The **Rh−** builds up antibodies (agglutinins) against **Rh+**.
Agglutination
There are no Rh agglutinogens in the donor blood.
Maternal type: **Rh−** Fetal type: **Rh+**

CHAPTER 12

Overview of the Heart

1. The **apex** of the heart is directed inferiorly and to the left.
About **2/3** of the heart mass is on the left side.
The heart is located in the **middle** mediastinum, between the second and **sixth** ribs.

2. 4 (epicardium)
1 (fibrous pericardium)
3 (pericardial cavity)
2 (parietal pericardium)

Structure of the Heart

1. Myocardium
Right atrium
Tricuspid
Endocardium
Left atrium
Fossa ovalis
Right ventricle
Trabeculae carneae
Bicuspid (mitral)
Aortic semilunar valve
Coronary arteries
Right atrium

2. M (right atrium)
Q (right ventricle)
F (left atrium)
I (left ventricle)
R (interventricular septum)
L (superior vena cava)
P (inferior vena cava)
E (pulmonary trunk)
C (ascending aorta)
K (right brachiocephalic vein)
J (brachiocephalic artery)
G (aortic semilunar valve)
N (pulmonary semilunar valve)
O (tricuspid valve)
H (bicuspid valve)
A (left common carotid artery)

B (left subclavian artery)
D (left pulmonary artery)
3. 13 (aortic semilunar valve)
14 (ascending aorta)
11 (bicuspid valve)
8 (capillaries of lungs)
10 (left atrium)
12 (left ventricle)
5 (pulmonary semilunar valve)
6 (pulmonary trunk)
9 (pulmonary veins)
7 (pulmonary arteries)
2 (right atrium)
4 (right ventricle)
3 (tricuspid valve)
1 (venae cavae)

Physiology of the Heart

1. Sinoatrial node
0.8 second
P wave
Sinoatrial node
Electrocardiogram
QRS wave
Systole
Conduction myofibers
T wave
Diastole
Atrioventricular bundle
0.1 second
Sinoatrial node
0.3 second

2. D (atria are in systole)
D (atrioventricular valves open)
S (atrioventricular valves close)
S (semilunar valves open)
D (semilunar valves close)
S (blood is ejected from the heart)
D (pressure in ventricles decreases)
D (blood enters ventricles)

3. (a) AV valves
(b) SL valves

4. False; <u>plus</u> should be times
True
False; <u>decreases</u> should be increases
False; <u>decreases</u> should be increases
True
True
False; <u>decreases</u> should be increases

True
True
False; <u>pons</u> should be medulla oblongata
False; <u>decreases</u> should be increases
True

CHAPTER 13

Classification and Structure of Blood Vessels

1. A (carries blood away ...)
C (functions in the exchange...)
C (wall consists of simple...)
V (carries blood toward heart)
V (has valves)
A (has three relatively thick...)
V (has three relatively thin...)
A (may have vasa vasorum)

2. (a) connective tissue–tunica externa
(b) simple squamous epithelium–tunica intima
(c) smooth muscle–tunica media

Physiology of Circulation

1. Diffusion
Diffusion
Osmosis
Filtration

2. V (osmotic pressure is greater...)
A (hydrostatic pressure is greater...)
A (net movement of fluid out...)
V (net movement of fluid into...)

3. Aorta
Capillary
Vein
Capillary
Artery
Blood pressure
Skeletal muscle contraction
Respiratory movements
Smooth muscle vasoconstriction
Systolic
Diastolic
Sphygmomanometer

Pulse pressure
Korotkoff sounds
Relaxes

4. A. Common carotid a.
    B. Brachial a.
    C. Radial a.
    D. Dorsalis pedis a.
    E. Temporal a.
    F. Facial a.
    G. Axillary a.
    H. Femoral a.

5. Medulla oblongata
    Cardiac center
    Vasomotor center
    Baroreceptors (pressorecep-
    tors)
    Chemoreceptors
    Renin
    Vasoconstriction
    Increase aldosterone
    Aldosterone

6. Checks for increase:
    A marked increase in blood
    volume
    An increase in heart rate
    Polycythemia
    Sympathetic stimulation of
    arterioles
    Production of angiotensin
    Checks for decrease:
    Loss of body fluids
    Vasodilation
    Slow heartbeat

Circulatory Pathways

1. Right atrium → **tricuspid
    valve** → right ventricle → **pul-
    monary semilunar valve** →
    pulmonary trunk → **pulmo-
    nary artery** → capillaries of
    lungs → **pulmonary veins** →
    left atrium.

2. A. Anterior cerebral a.
    B. Internal carotid a.
    C. Posterior communicating
        a.
    D. Basilar a.
    E. Middle cerebral a.
    F. Posterior cerebral a.
    G. Vertebral a.

3. Coronary a.
    Brachiocephalic a.
    Left subclavian a.
    Common carotid a.
    Vertebral a.
    Left common carotid a.

4. Brachial a.

Radial a.
Ulnar a.
Common hepatic a.
Left gastric a.
Splenic a.
Superior mesenteric a.
Renal a.
Inferior mesenteric a.
Common iliac a.
Internal iliac a.
Femoral a.
Popliteal a.
Posterior tibial a.
Anterior tibial a.

5. Inferior vena cava
    Superior vena cava
    Right and left brachiocephalic
    v.
    Internal jugular v.
    Basilic v.
    Cephalic v.
    Median cubital v.
    Brachial v.
    Azygos v.
    Hepatic v.
    Hepatic portal v.
    Splenic v.
    Superior mesenteric v.
    Great saphenous v.
    Common iliac v.
    Internal iliac v.
    Femoral v.
    Anterior tibial v.
    Posterior tibial v.

6. Umbilical artery
    Umbilical vein
    Ductus venosus
    Foramen ovale
    Ductus arteriosus
    Placenta

7. Left ventricle → aortic semilu-
    nar valve → **ascending aorta**
    → aortic arch → **brachioce-
    phalic artery** → **right com-
    mon carotid artery** → **right
    internal carotid artery** →
    right middle cerebral artery.

8. Left gonad → left gonadal vein
    → **left renal vein** → **IVC** →
    right atrium → **tricuspid**
    valve → **right ventricle** →
    pulmonary semilunar valve
    → **pulmonary trunk** → **pul-
    monary artery** → capillaries
    of lungs → **pulmonary vein**
    → **left atrium** → **bicuspid**

valve → **left ventricle** →
aortic semilunar valve →
ascending aorta → aortic arch
→ **left subclavian artery** →
left axillary artery → **left
brachial artery** → **left radial
artery** → capillaries on lateral
side of left forearm.

9. Descending aorta → **celiac
    trunk** → **splenic artery** →
    capillaries of the spleen →
    splenic vein → **hepatic por-
    tal vein** → sinusoids of liver →
    hepatic vein → **IVC** → right
    atrium.

CHAPTER 14

Functions of the Lymphatic System

1. Return excess interstitial fluid
    to the blood
    Absorption of fats and fat solu-
    ble vitamins
    Defense against invading
    microorganisms

Components of the Lymphatic System

1. Lymph
    Lymphatic vessels
    Lymphatic organs

2. Interstitial fluid
    Blood plasma
    Lymph
    Interstitial fluid
    Lymph capillaries
    Lymphatic ducts
    Right lymphatic duct
    Thoracic duct
    Cisterna chyli
    Right lymphatic duct
    Thoracic duct
    Valves
    Skeletal muscle action
    Respiratory movements
    Contraction of smooth muscle
    in vessel walls

3. Lymphocytes
    Lymph nodes
    Tonsils
    Spleen
    Thymus
    Lymph nodes
    Spleen
    Tonsils (pharyngeal)
    Thymus

Spleen
Tonsils (pharyngeal)
Afferent lymphatic vessel
Thymosin
Spleen

Resistance to Disease

1. Pathogens
Resistance
Susceptibility
Nonspecific mechanisms
Specific mechanisms
Immunity
2. Leukocytosis
Fever
Decrease in blood pressure
3. A   (unbroken skin and mucous membranes)
B   (activates phagocytosis and inflammation)
B   (blocks replication of viruses)
A   (cilia action in respiratory tract)
B   (interferon)
D   (accompanied by swelling, heat, redness)
C   (ingestion and digestion of solid particles)
B   (action of complement)
C   (macrophages and neutrophils)
D   (aimed at localizing damage)
4. Specificity
Memory
Lymphocytes
Macrophages
Antigens
T-lymphocytes (T-cells)
B-lymphocytes (B-cells)
T-cells
B-cells
B-cells
T-cells
Plasma cells
Immunoglobulins
Primary response
Killer T-cells
Helper T-cells
Suppressor T-cells
Memory T-cells
Plasma cells
Memory B-cells
5. IgG (most numerous antibody)
IgE (responsible for allergies)

IgA (found in breast milk, saliva)
IgM (responsible for ABO reactions)
IgG (major antibody in immune response)
IgE (binds to mast cells)
IgG (crosses placenta)
IgM (causes agglutination of antigens)
6. D   (antiserum is injected…)
A   (a person contracts a disease…)
C   (antibodies are transferred…)
B   (antigens deliberately introduced…)
A   (memory cells …)
D   (antibodies injected…)
C   (IgA antibodies in mother's milk)
B   (mumps, diphtheria…vaccines)

CHAPTER 15

Functions and Overview of Respiration

1. Ventilation
External respiration
Transport
Internal respiration
Cellular respiration

Ventilation

1. L   (bronchi)
U   (nose)
U   (larynx)
U   (pharynx)
L   (lungs)
L   (trachea)
2. Warm the air
Filter the air
Moisten the air
Nasopharynx
Nasopharynx
Oropharynx
Laryngopharynx
Thyroid
Cricoid
Epiglottis
Glottis (rima glottis)
Trachea
Carina
Pseudostratified ciliated columnar epithelium
Simple squamous epithelium

3. 6   (alveolar ducts)
5   (respiratory bronchioles)
7   (alveoli)
3   (segmental bronchi)
2   (lobar bronchi)
4   (terminal bronchioles)
1   (primary bronchi)
4. L   (cardiac notch)
L   (two lobes)
R   (shorter and wider)
B   (divided into lobules)
B   (rests on the diaphragm)
R   (has two fissures)
B   (enclosed by pleura)
B   (anchored at the root or hilum)
5. Intrapleural pressure
Atmospheric pressure
Intrapulmonary pressure
Intrapleural pressure
Diaphragm
Internal intercostals
Surfactant
Spirometer
Intrapulmonary pressure
Atmospheric pressure
6. I   (diaphragm contracts)
E   (intrapulmonary exceeds atmospheric)
I   (external intercostal muscles may contract)
I   (atmospheric greater than intrapulmonary)
I   (lung volume increases)
E   (diaphragm relaxes)
E   (internal intercostal muscles may contract)
I   (air flows into the lungs)
E   (elastic recoil decreases size of alveoli)
7. IC = Inspiratory capacity
TV = Tidal volume
FRC = Functional residual capacity
VC = Vital capacity
IRV = Inspiratory reserve volume
TLC = Total lung capacity
ERV = Expiratory reserve volume
FRC = Functional residual capacity
RV = Residual volume
TLC = Total lung capacity
8. First row: TLC = 5700 ml; VC = 4500 ml

Second row: TV = 600 ml; RV = 1000 ml

Third row: TLC = 5800 ml; IRV = 3300 ml

Fourth row: ERV = 1200 ml; RV = 1300 ml

9. Young adults > (greater than)
Females < (less than)
Short people < (less than)
Normal weight people > (greater than)
Healthy people > (greater than)
Good physical condition > (greater than)

Basic Gas Laws and Respiration

1. 21% × 750 mm Hg = 157.5 mm Hg
2. Solubility of each gas and partial pressures
3. External respiration is the exchange of gases between the **alveoli in the lungs and the blood in the capillaries**. Internal respiration is the exchange of gases between the **blood in the capillaries and the tissue cells**.
4. (a) Fluid that lines the alveolus
   (b) Simple squamous epith. of alveolar wall
   (c) Basement membrane of epith.
   (d) Interstitial space
   (e) Basement membrane of capillary epith.
   (f) Simple squamous epith. of capillary wall
5. D
   D
   I
   D

Transport of Gases

1. Dissolved in plasma
   Bound to hemoglobin as oxyhemoglobin
2. Dissolved in plasma
   Bound to Hb as carbaminohemoglobin
   As bicarbonate ions in plasma
3. Oxyhemoglobin
   Bicarbonate ions
   Carbaminohemoglobin
   Carbonic acid

Carbonic anhydrase

4. Should have checks (√) before the following:
Increased partial pressure of carbon dioxide
Increased hydrogen ion concentration
Increased temperature
Increased cellular metabolism

5. E (oxygen diffuses into blood)
I (oxygen diffuses out of blood)
I (carbon dioxide diffuses into blood)
E (carbon dioxide diffuses out of blood)
E (occurs in alveolus)
I (occurs in body tissues)
I (bicarbonate ion is formed)
E (bicarbonate ions release carbon dioxide)
E (oxyhemoglobin is formed)
I (oxyhemoglobin dissociates)

Regulation of Respiration

1. The respiratory center includes neurons in the **pons** and **medulla oblongata**.
2. The inspiratory areas of the respiratory center send impulses along the **phrenic** nerve to the diaphragm and along the **intercostal** nerves to the external intercostal muscles.
3. F (Chemoreceptors in the medulla…)
T (Increases in blood…)
T (Increases in hydrogen ion…)
T (Chemoreceptors in the medulla…)
F (A decrease in oxygen…)
T (Decreased oxygen levels…)
T (Peripheral chemoreceptors…)
T (The Hering-Breuer reflex prevents…)
T (The Hering-Breuer reflex is…)
F (Higher brain centers…)
F (Anxiety decreases…)

T (Chronic pain stimulates…)
F (Decreasing body temperature…)
T (The primary stimulus…)

CHAPTER 16

Introduction

1. G (esophagus)
H (gallbladder)
J (large intestine)
I (liver)
F (mouth)
D (pancreas)
B (pharynx)
A (salivary gland)
E (small intestine)
C (stomach)
There should be an asterisk by each accessory organ, H, I, D, and A.

Functions of the Digestive System

1. Mastication
Hydrolysis
Chemical digestion
Deglutition
Peristalsis
Absorption
Defecation

General Structure of the Digestive Tract

1. A (Innermost layer…)
C (Contains blood…)
B (Responsible for most…)
A (Consists of simple…)
B (Contains inner …)
C (Contains Meissner's…)
B (Contains the myenteric…)

Components of the Digestive Tract

1. Buccinator
Palate
Uvula
Lingual tonsils
Papillae
Incisors
Canines
Parotid
Submandibular
Salivary amylase
Cleansing action on teeth
Moistens and lubricates food

Dissolves molecules for taste

Begins chemical digestion of carbohydrates

2. G (Alveolar process)
   D (Apical foramen)
   C (Cementum)
   E (Dentin)
   A (Enamel)
   B (Gingiva)
   F (Pulp cavity)
   H (Root canal)
3. Fauces
   Nasopharynx
   Nasopharynx
   Oropharynx
   Uvula
   Epiglottis
   Esophagus
   Esophageal hiatus
   Lower esophageal or cardiac
4. C (Body)
   B (Cardiac region)
   H (Duodenum)
   A (Fundus)
   F (Lower esophageal sphincter)
   G (Pyloric sphincter)
   E (Pylorus)
   D (Rugae)
5. Hydrochloric acid
   Gastrin
   Pepsin
   Chyme
   Absorption of vitamin B_{12}
   Receptivity of duodenum
   Nature of contents (fluidity of chyme)
6. C (Triggered by…)
   A (Begins with thoughts…)
   B (Begins when food…)
   C (Inhibits gastric secretions)
   B (Involves distention…)
7. Duodenum
   Plicae circulares
   Villi
   Microvilli
   Lacteal
   Duodenum
   Ileum
   Enterokinase
   Cholecystokinin
   Secretin
   Lipase
   Cholecystokinin (pancreozymin)
   Chyme in small intestine

8. Absorption of water and electrolytes
   Removal of waste materials
9. H (Where small…)
   L (Three bands…)
   E (Pieces of fat…)
   C (Blind pouch that…)
   B (Portion of large…)
   G (Right colonic flexure)
   K (Left colonic flexure)
   M (Portion of large intestine between…)
   D (Portion of large intestine on the left…)
   J (S-shaped curve…)
   I (Portion that follows…)
   A (Terminal opening…)
   F (Series of pouches…)

Accessory Organs of Digestion

1. Falciform ligament
   Caudate lobe
   Quadrate lobe
   Liver lobule
   Sinusoids
   Hepatic artery
   Hepatic portal vein
   Hepatic vein
   Bile
   Bilirubin
   Emulsify fats
   Gallbladder
   Cystic duct
   Cholecystokinin
   Common bile duct
   Hepatic artery
   Hepatic portal vein
   Hepatic duct
2. Pancreatic islets (of Langerhans)
   Acinar cells
   Pancreatic duct (of Wirsung)
   Pancreatic amylase
   Trypsin
   Lipase
   Secretin
   Cholecystokinin (pancreozymin)

Chemical Digestion

1. Row 1: Amylase
   Row 2: Maltase, small intestine
   Row 3: Small intestine, sucrose to fructose and glucose
   Row 4: Lactase, small intestine
   Row 5: Pepsin
   Row 6: Pancreas

   Row 7: Peptidase, pancreas
   Row 8: Lipase, pancreas
2. Glucose, fructose, galactose
3. Amino acids
4. Monoglycerides and fatty acids

Absorption

1. Blood capillary
   Lacteal
   Micelles
   Chylomicron
   Chyle
2. Active transport
   Facilitated diffusion
   Osmosis
   Simple diffusion

CHAPTER 17

Metabolism of Absorbed Nutrients

1. Metabolism
   Cellular metabolism
   Enzymes
   Nutrition
2. H (Most important simple sugar…)
   C (Term that means…)
   L (Reactions in which glucose is…)
   M (Fate of pyruvic acid…)
   B (Term that means…)
   A (Molecule that enters…)
   I (Storage form of glucose)
   E (Location of glycolysis reactions)
   O (Location of citric…)
   J (Conversion of glucose to glycogen)
   N (Conversion of glucose to fat)
   K (Conversion of glycogen into glucose)
   G (Conversion of noncarbohydrate…)
   F (Principal reaction…)
   D (Reactions that convert…)
3. Build new tissues
   Replace damaged tissues
   Synthesis of hemoglobin
   Synthesis of enzymes
   Synthesis of hormones
   Synthesis of plasma proteins
4. Acetyl-CoA
   Pyruvic acid
5. A calorie is the amount of heat required to raise the tempera-

ture of one kilogram of water one degree Celsius, from 14° to 15°.

6. Basal metabolism
Physical activity
Thermogenesis
Basal metabolism accounts for most of the energy used and physical activity is the one that can be controlled voluntarily.

Basic Elements of Nutrition
1. C (Primary energy source)
P (Regulate body processes)
L (Major component of cell membranes)
L (Transport vitamins A, D, E, K)
C (Add bulk to the diet)
L (Fatty acids)
L (Provide insulation and protection)
P (Provide structure)
C (Glucose)
L (Concentrated energy)
C (Fiber)
P (Hormones, enzymes)
L (Steroids)
C (Glycogen)
L (Triglycerides)
P (Amino acids)
2. 4 (1 gram pure carbohydrate)
4 (1 gram pure protein)
9 (1 gram pure fat)
20 (5 grams carbohydrate)
16 (4 grams protein)
27 (3 grams fat)
3. Amino acids that cannot be synthesized in the body and must be supplied in the diet are called **essential** amino acids. A protein that contains all of these amino acids is called a **complete** protein. Other proteins, called incomplete proteins should be eaten in combinations to provide all of the **essential** amino acids.
4. The American Heart Association recommends that no more than **30 percent** of the daily calorie intake should be in the form of fats. Further, it recommends a reduction in the amount of saturated fats in the diet. In general, foods

that are high in saturated fats are also high in **cholesterol**. Cholesterol intake should be limited to less than **250 mg** per day.
5. W (Thiamine)
W (Niacin)
F (Vitamin A)
W (Vitamin C)
F (Vitamin D)
W (Riboflavin)
6. W (Medium for chemical reactions)
V (Release energy from nutrients)
V (Nucleic acid synthesis)
M (Incorporated into bones and teeth)
W (Maintenance of body temperature)
W (Regulation of body fluid levels)

Body Temperature
1. E (Byproduct…)
F (Location…)
C (Temperature…)
D (Heat…)
A (Distributes…)
J [Methods of increasing body heat (2)]
B
H (Methods of releasing body heat)
G
I (Temperature…)

CHAPTER 18
Components of the Urinary System
1. Rids the body of wastes
Regulates fluid volume
Maintains electrolyte concentration
Controls blood pH
Secretes erythropoietin
Secretes renin
2. Kidney, ureter, bladder, urethra.
3. D Major calyx
B Minor calyx
A Renal capsule
I Renal column
H Renal cortex
F Renal papilla
C Renal pelvis

G Renal pyramid
E Ureter
4. B Afferent arteriole
E Ascending limb
D Collecting duct
J Descending limb
C Distal convoluted tubule
A Efferent arteriole
H Glomerular capsule
I Glomerulus
F Nephron loop
G Proximal convoluted tubule
5. Macula densa
Juxtaglomerular cells
Renin
Macula densa
1200 ml/minute
Segmental arteries
Interlobar artery
Arcuate artery
Interlobular artery
Afferent arteriole
Peritubular capillaries
Renal column
Segmental veins
6. Ureters
Transitional
Urinary bladder
Rugae
Transitional
Detrusor
Trigone
Smooth (involuntary)
Skeletal (voluntary)
Urethra
Prostatic urethra
Spongy (penile) urethra

Urine Formation
1. C (Tubular cells to filtrate)
A (Glomerulus to capsule)
B (Tubules to capillaries)
2. Blue circles around GOP and CHP.
Red circle around GHP.
Net filtration pressure = 10 mm Hg. (GHP – GOP – CHP)
3. Aldosterone
Antidiuretic hormone
Atrial natriuretic hormone (atriopeptin)
Renin
Angiotensin
Micturition
4. 1) Decreases or reduces
2) Osmosis

3) Active transport
4) Carrier molecules
5) Threshold
6) Urine (filtrate)
7) Secretion
8) Hydrogen

5. It is a powerful vasoconstrictor.
   It increases aldosterone, which increases sodium and water reabsorption to increase blood volume, which increases blood pressure.

Characteristics of Urine

1. Checks (√) before the following:
   The color of urine is due to urochrome.
   Urine is usually slightly acidic,...
   High protein diets tend to make...
   The specific gravity of urine...
   The predominant solute in urine is urea.
2. Pyuria (White blood cells)
   Albuminuria (Albumin)
   Glucosuria (Glucose)
   Hematuria (Erythrocytes)

Body Fluids

1. Beverages (* most)
   Food
   Metabolic water
2. Urine (* most)
   Lungs
   Skin
   GI tract
3. D   20 percent (Extracellular)
   E   15–16 percent (Interstitial)
   C   40 percent (Intracellular)
   F   4–5 percent (Plasma)
   A   40 percent (Solutes)
   B   60 percent (Total fluids)
4. Sodium
   Chloride
   Potassium
   Phosphates
   Aldosterone
5. 7.35–7.45
   Alkalosis
   Acidosis
   Buffers
   Respiratory system
   Kidneys

CHAPTER 19

Male Reproductive System

1. D   (Bulbourethral gland)
   M   (Corpus cavernosum)
   E   (Corpus spongiosum)
   F   (Ductus deferens)
   C   (Ejaculatory duct)
   L   (Epididymis)
   N   (Glans penis)
   J   (Prostate)
   H   (Scrotum)
   I   (Symphysis pubis)
   G   (Testicle)
   B   (Urethra)
   K   (Urethra)
   A   (Urinary bladder)
2. 6   (Ductus deferens)
   4   (Efferent ducts)
   7   (Ejaculatory duct)
   5   (Epididymis)
   9   (Membranous urethra)
   10 (Penile urethra)
   8   (Prostatic urethra)
   3   (Rete testis)
   1   (Seminiferous tubules)
   2   (Straight tubules)
3. Testes
   Spermatozoa (sperm)
   Scrotum
   Dartos
   Cremaster
   Tunica albuginea
   Seminiferous tubules
   Interstitial cells
   Spermiogenesis
   Midpiece (neck)
   23
   Supporting cells (Sertoli)
4. C   (Product secreted...)
   B   (Encircles...)
   A   (Located posterior...)
   A   (Secretion accounts...)
   C   (Located near...)
   C   (Smallest of...)
   A   (Secretion has...)
5. 1. Parasympathetic
   2. Arteries
   3. Veins
   4. Erection
   5. Sympathetic
   6. Emission
   7. Ejaculation
   8. Increased
   9. Increased
   10. Increased respiration
   11. Orgasm or climax

6. GnRH
   Testosterone
   LH or ICSH
   Androgens
   FSH
   LH
   FSH
   Adrenal cortex
   Spermatogenesis
   Development and maintenance of secondary sex characteristics

Female Reproductive System

1. I   (Cervix)
   G   (Clitoris)
   H   (Infundibulum)
   F   (Mons pubis)
   A   (Ovary)
   J   (Rectum)
   E   (Symphysis pubis)
   L   (Urethra)
   D   (Urinary bladder)
   B   (Uterine tube)
   C   (Uterus)
   K   (Vagina)
2. Ovary
   Primary oocyte
   Secondary oocyte
   Zona pellucida
   Corona radiata
   Corpus luteum
   Fimbriae
   External os
   Broad ligament
   Myometrium
   Stratum functionale
   Hymen
3. D   (Antrum)
   J   (Corpus albicans)
   I   (Corpus luteum)
   G   (Fimbriae)
   A   (Infundibulum)
   F   (Primary follicle)
   E   (Secondary follicle)
   B   (Secondary oocyte)
   H   (Uterine tube)
   C   (Vesicular follicle)
4. Vulva or pudendum
   Labia majora
   Mons pubis
   Vestibule
   Clitoris
   Paraurethral glands
   Greater vestibular glands
5. True (The female...)

False (Sympathetic responses...)

True (Sympathetic responses...)

6. A (Starts the events...)

B, C (Levels increase...)

A (Secreted by hypothalamus)

B, C (Secreted by anterior pituitary)

C (Triggers ovulation)

D, E (Secreted by corpus luteum)

D (Secreted by cells...)

E (Stimulates secretory phase...)

D (Stimulates proliferative...)

C (Stimulates development of the corpus luteum)

D (Stimulates development of glandular...)

E (Stimulates development of the duct...)

D (Causes an accumulation...)

B (Stimulates growth...)

D, E (Levels decrease...)

7. Increases

Increases

Increases

Decreases

Decreases

8. Areola

Suspensory (Cooper's) ligaments

Lactiferous duct

Lactiferous sinus (ampulla)

Prolactin

Oxytocin

CHAPTER 20

Fertilization

1. Zygote

Corona radiata

Capacitation

24 hours

Uterine tube

Preembryonic Period

1. Cleavage

Implantation

Formation of germ layers

Cleavage

Blastomeres

Morula

Blastocyst

Inner cell mass

Blastocele

Trophoblast

Chorion

Stratum functionale of endometrium

Human chorionic gonadotropin (HCG)

Progesterone

Inner cell mass

Ectoderm

Mesoderm

Endoderm

Embryonic Development

1. The period of embryonic development lasts from the beginning of the **third** week after conception to the end of the **eighth** week. Three significant developments during this period are the formation of the **extraembryonic** membranes, formation of the **placenta**, and formation of all the body **organ** systems. During this period the developing offspring is called an **embryo**.

2. A   (Forms a sac...)

D   (Produces the primordial...)

B   (Becomes part...)

C   (Develops from...)

A   (Cushions and protects...)

C   (Contributes to...)

C   (Develops fingerlike...)

A   (Filled with fluid)

3. 1. Chorionic villi

2. Endometrium

3. Chorionic villi

4. Umbilical

5. Blood

6. Oxygen

7. Carbon dioxide

8. Fetal blood

9. Maternal blood

4. C   (Epithelial lining the digestive tract)

A   (Epidermis of the skin)

B   (Cardiac muscle)

A   (Nervous tissue)

B   (Cartilage)

A   (Hair, nails, glands of the skin)

C   (Respiratory epithelium)

B   (Epithelium lining the blood vessels)

A   (Lining of the oral cavity)

B   (Bone)

B   (Dermis of the skin)

A   (Epithelial lining of the vagina)

Fetal Development

1. Quickening

Vernix caseosa

Lanugo hair

Foramen ovale

Umbilical vein

Ductus venosus

Parturition and Lactation

1. Parturition

Labor

Progesterone

Estrogen

Posterior pituitary gland

Prostaglandins

Positive feedback

Dilation stage

Expulsion stage

Dilation stage

Placental stage

Cephalic (head first)

2. 1. Collapsed

2. Umbilical cord

3. Carbon dioxide

4. pH (acidosis)

5. Decreasing

6. Medulla

3. Lactation

Prolactin

Oxytocin

Estrogen

Progesterone

Colostrum

4. 1. Hypothalamus

2. Prolactin releasing hormone

3. Prolactin

4. Milk production

5. Ceases

6. Days

Postnatal Development

1. Neonatal

Senescence

Childhood

Infancy

Adolescence

Infancy

Childhood

Senescence

Answers to Using Clinical Knowledge

CHAPTER 1

1. C (Evidence of disease that can …)
   A (Name of a disease …)
   B (Prediction of the course …)
   D (A combination of signs …)
   E (Evidence of disease that can only be …)
2. DOB = date of birth
   H&P = history and physical
   BP = blood pressure
   Dx = diagnosis
   ac = before meals
   prn = as needed
   qid = four times a day
   IV = intravenous
   mg = milligram
   ant = anterior
3. A check mark should be before: homeostasis, prognosis, visceral, hypochondriac
   saggital should be sagittal
   endocryn should be endocrine
   phyziology should be physiology
   epinime should be eponym
   limfatic should be lymphatic
   addominopelvic should be abdominopelvic
4. Visceral (pertaining to internal organs)
   Cardiography (process of making a recording of the heart)
   Gastrology (study of the stomach)
   Dorsal (pertaining to the back)
   Pathology (study of disease)

CHAPTER 2

1. F (Nonproprietary drug name …)
   D (Presence of a disease in a given…)
   E (Study of causes of diseases)
   B (Alpha-methyl-4 …)
   G (An illness that occurs without …)
   C (Smallest unit is a molecule)
   A (Drug name that is assigned by …)
   H (An infection acquired from …)
   J (The water in a normal saline solution)
   I (A widespread epidemic …)
2. CHO = carbohydrate
   VS = vital signs
   ADL = activities of daily living
   stat = immediately
   Px = prognosis
3. A check mark should be before: covalent, iatrogenic
   proteen should be protein
   asid should be acid
   element should be element
4. calor = heat
   tetr = four
   aer = air, gas
   hydro = water; lys = to take apart
   pent = five
   alkal = basic
   lact = milk
   sacchar = sugar or sweet
   lip = fat
   gluc = sweetness or sugar

CHAPTER 3

1. B (Loss of differentiation in cells …)
   K (The route used when administering …)
   J (RBCs shrink when placed …)
   E (Enlargement of an organ due …)
   M (Process by which a cell may …)
   H (Death of a group of cells)
   I (Any new or abnormal growth …)
   A (It takes cellular energy to move…)
   C (Not malignant; not recurring)

   F (Type of cell division ….)
2. DNA = deoxyribonucleic acid
   PBI = protein-bound iodine
   LBW = low birth rate
   NB = newborn
   NPO = nothing by mouth
3. A check mark should be before: meiosis, cytokinesis
   benine should be benign
   anomoly should be anomaly
   displasia should be dysplasia
4. cyto = cell
   phag = to eat, devour
   tonic = solute strength
   som = body
   reti = network, lattice
5. ic = pertaining to
   elle = little, small
   osis = condition of
   itis = inflammation of
   al = pertaining to

CHAPTER 4

1. I (Study that involves…)
   D (Tumor derived from fat cells)
   A (Abnormal joining of …)
   F (Cells that release …)
   B (Removal and microscopic …)
   G (Study of the structural...)
   J (Malignant growth derived from connective …)
   C (Malignant growth derived fore epithelial…)
2. D5W = 5% dextrose in water
   NS = normal saline
   IM = intramuscular
   tiw = three times a week
   ASA = aspirin
3. A check mark should be before: macrophage, neuroglia, papilloma
   skurvy should be scurvy
   condrocyte should be chondrocyte
4. vacu = empty
   auscult = listen

cohes = stick together
strict = narrowing
adip = fat
strat = layer
inocul = implant, introduce
5. macro = large
    pseudo = false
    multi = many
    blast = to form, sprout
    oma = tumor, swelling, mass
    aden = gland
    neur = nerve
    glia = glue
    eryth = red
    squam = flattened, scaly

CHAPTER 5

1. C (Deepest layer of skin …)
    A (Baldness)
    G (Sunscreen preparations)
    E (A slough produced by …)
    H (Severe itching)
    F (A mole)
    B (Inflammation of the skin)
    J (Hives)
2. UV = ultraviolet
    EAHF = eczema, asthma, and
    hay fever
    ung = ointment
    HSV = herpes simplex virus
    I&D = incision and drainage
3. A check mark should be
    before: eczema, impetigo, sub-
    cutaneous
    carotinization should be kerati-
    nization
    sebacious should be sebaceous
4. cer = wax
    sud = sweat
    ichthy = scaly, dry
    onych = nail
    ectomy = surgical incision
    plasty = surgical repair
    xer = dry
    cidal = killing
    cyan = blue
    pedicu = louse or lice
5. hidr = sweat, aden = gland,
    itis = inflammation or infec-
    tion
    hidradenitis = inflammation of
    a sweat gland
    myco = fungus, dermat =
    skin, itis = inflammation or
    infection

mycodermatitis = fungal infection of the skin

CHAPTER 6

1. C (Shaft of a long bone)
    E (Uric acid crystals
    develop …)
    G (Bone forming cell)
    K (Congenital deformity of the
    foot …)
    F (Ibuprofen)
    D (Displacement of a bone …)
    B (Inflammation of a joint)
    I (Twisting of a joint …)
    L (Acetominophen)
    A (Slightly movable joint)
2. DJD = degenerative joint dis-
    ease
    CTS = carpal tunnel syndrome
    ROM = range of motion
    fx = fracture
    DIPJ = distal interphalangeal
    joint
3. symarthrosis should be synar-
    throsis
    ileum should be ilium (ileum
    is from the digestive system)
    carpel should be carpal
    fibia should be tibia (or fibula)
    falanges should be phalanges
4. kyph = hump
    poie = formation or making
    spondy = vertebrae
    arthr = joint
    myel = bone marrow
5. phalangectomy = Excision of a
    finger or toe
    costalgia = Pain in the ribs
    chondropathy = Disease of
    cartilage
    arthectomy = Surgical removal
    of a joint
    osteoarthropathy = Any dis-
    ease of both bones and joints
6. osteo = bone, plasty = surgi-
    cal repair
    osteoplasty means surgical
    repair of a bone
    ankly = crooked, bent, or stiff,
    osis = condition of
    ankylosis means immobility of
    a joint

CHAPTER 7

1. C (Slight muscle paralysis)

B (Inflammation of a fascia)
D (Muscle disease)
F (Inflammation of a muscle)
I (Suture of a tendon)
J (Spasmodic involuntary
twitching …)
A (Painful involuntary muscle
spasm)
2. ACL = anterior cruciate liga-
    ment
    LOS = length of stay
    RSI = repetitive stress injury
    PMA = progressive muscular
    atrophy
    DTR = deep tendon reflex
3. (myosin)   mysin
    myorexis   (myorrhexis)
    diaphram   (diaphragm)
    (acetylcholine)   acetilcoline
    gastronemius   (gastrocne-
                      mius)
    (aponeurosis)   apronuro-
                      sis
4. myopathy = Any abnormal
    condition …
    fasciorraphy = Suturing of
    torn fascia
    myotomy = Surgical incision
    into…
    fasciodesis = Suture of a fascia
    to …
    myoplasty = surgical repair of
    a muscle
5. (a) Central-acting drugs
    depress the motor pathways in
    the brain stem and spinal cord,
    which decreases muscle tone.
    (b) lethargy, drowsiness, diz-
    ziness, confusion, headache,
    blurred vision

CHAPTER 8

1. D (Used in the treatment of
    migraine …)
    G (White, fatty substance
    around …)
    C (Antiparkinsonism agent)
    B (Lou Gehrig's disease)
    A (Nerve impulse)
    H (Occipital lobe)
    J (Painful disorder …)
    I (Contains pneumotaxic …)
2. CVA = cerebrovascular acci-
    dent
    EEG = electroencephalogram
    CSF = cerebrospinal fluid

ADD = attention deficit disorder

CT = computed tomography

3. (synapse) sinapse
ponds (pons)
neurolemma (neurilemma)
(sclerosis) sclairosis
triginal (trigeminal)

4. schiz = division or split
lepsy = seizure
narc = numbness or stupor or sleep
alges = relationship to pain
gloss = tongue
plex = network or interweave
mening = membrane
esthes = feeling

5. encephalitis = Inflammation of the brain
neuroplasty = Surgical repair of a nerve
myelitis = Inflammation of the spinal cord
encephalopathy = Any degenerative disease of the brain
myelogram = Record of a study of the spinal cord

CHAPTER 9

1. G (Cause pupil dilation)
H (Responds to tissue damage)
E (Inflammation of the inner ear)
M (Impairment of hearing …)
B (Paralyze ciliary muscle …)
K (Fungal infection of …)
I (Night blindness)
N (Ringing or buzzing sound…)
A (Defective curvature of …)
D (Characterized by increased …)

2. REM = Rapid eye movement
EOM = Extraocular movement
EENT = Eye, ear, nose, throat
OS = Left eye (oculus sinister)
AD = Right ear (auris dexter)

3. A check mark should be before: eustachian, lacrimal
oldfactory should be olfactory
gustatary should be gustatory
retna should be retina

4. blephar = eyelid
opia = visual condition
pha = lens of the eye
myring = tympanic membrane

lith = stone, calculus

5. iridectomy = Excision of a full-thickness…
keratotomy = Incision of the cornea
otoplasty = Plastic surgery of the external ear
myringectomy = Excision of the tympanic …
dacryoma = Tumorlike swelling due to …

CHAPTER 10

1. L (Synthetic glucocorticoid)
M (Derived from arachidonic …)
N (Premature aging that occurs …)
E (Caused by a deficient …)
G (Used to treat decreased …)
J (Excessive thirst)
A (Caused by excessive growth …)
I (Posterior portion of …)
C (Tumor of a gland)
D (A group of symptoms …)

2. ACTH = adrenocorticotropic hormone
ADH = antidiuretic hormone
DKA = diabetic ketoacidosis
FSH = follicle-stimulating hormone
IDDM = insulin-dependent diabetes mellitus

3. epinefrin should be epinephrine
hydrocloric should be hydrochloric
natrietic should be natriuretic
prostraglandins should be prostaglandins
lutinizing should be luteinizing

4. andr = male or maleness
crine = to secrete
gest = to carry (pregnancy)
pin = pinecone
toc = birth
acr = extremities
megaly = enlargement
ren = kidney
ad = toward
para = beside

5. F (Inflammation of the pancreas)
D (Surgical removal of the pituitary…)

G (Tumor of the pineal gland)
C (Any disorder of …)
A (Surgical removal of …)
B (Inflammation of the …)
E (Pain in the pancreas)
H (Enlargement of …)

CHAPTER 11

1. B (On the surface of RBCs)
F (Stem cell in the bone …)
L (Blood clot)
J (Multiple pinpoint …)
I (An increase in number…)
H (Malignant tumor of bone…)
E (Percentage of RBCs …)
K (Immature RBC)
C (Replace clotting factors …)
D (Oral anticoagulant …)

2. CBC = complete blood count
PCV = packed cell volume
Hb = hemoglobin
HCT = hematocrit
Rh = rhesus factor in blood

3. dipedesis should be diapedesis
lukosites should be leukocytes
hemopoesis should be hemopoiesia
agllutination should be agglutination
hemolitic should be hemolytic

4. eryth = red
kary = nucleus
throm = clot
mega = large
cyte = cell
penia = lack of or deficiency
poie = formation of
phil = affinity for
stasis = control
agglutin = clumping

CHAPTER 12

1. N (Contraction phase …)
F (Enlargement of the heart)
J (Rapid, random, irregular …)
G (Any primary disease …)
I (Drug that increases …)
M (Volume of blood ejected …)
C (Using a stethoscope …)
A (Acute chest pain …)
K (A vasodilator to relieve …)
L (Valves between the …)

2. CABG = coronary artery bypass graft
   PVC = premature ventricular contraction
   CPR = cardiopulmonary resuscitation
   VSD = ventricular septal defect
   CHF = congestive heart failure
3. arhythmia should be arrhythmia
   infarcshun should be infarction
   distole should diastole
   conjestive should be congestive
   fosa ovalis should be fossa ovalis
4. cardi = heart
   myo = muscle
   sten = narrowing
   tachy = rapid
   gram = recording or record
   lun = moon shaped
   sphyg = pulse
   coron = crown
   echo = sound
   steth = chest

CHAPTER 13

1. H (Sounds heard in …)
   L (Increase in size …)
   C (A calcium-channel blocker …)
   F (Varicose veins in …)
   J (Inflammation of veins)
   I (Opposition to blood flow)
   D (A diuretic used to …)
   A (Surgical repair of …)
   E (A benign tumor of …)
   G (Deficiency in blood supply …)
2. CVP = central venous pressure
   DSA = digital subtraction angiography
   KVO = keep vein open
   PTCA = percutaneous transluminal coronary angioplasty
   H&H = hemoglobin and hematocrit
3. sfincters should be sphincters
   distolic should be diastolic
   sphygmanometer should be sphygmomanometer
   peracardial should be pericardial
   aneurism should be aneurysm

4. ather = yellow fatty plaque
   isch = deficiency
   brach = arm
   ven = vein
   vas = vessel
   sten = narrowing or constriction
   scler = hard
   cephal = head
5. angiodermatitis = Inflammation of blood vessels in the skin
   phlebectomy = Surgical excision of a vein
   angiitis = Inflammation of any blood vessel
   arteriectomy = Surgical excision of an artery
   thrombophlebitis = Inflammation of a vein associated with…

CHAPTER 14

1. C (A substance that triggers …)
   J (Immunity produces when …)
   F (Used to reduce rejection …)
   I (Specialist in the diagnosis …)
   G (Malignant tumor of lymph nodes …)
   K (Ability to counteract the effects …)
   N (Detoxified antigenic agents …)
   A (An exaggerated or unusual …)
   H (Spread of a tumor to …)
   L (Enlargement of the spleen)
2. AIDS = acquired immunodeficiency syndrome
   CMV = cytomegalovirus
   KS = Kaposi's sarcoma
   HIV = human immunodeficiency virus
   IDC = invasive ductal carcinoma
3. A check mark should be before: immunoglobulins, vaccination, pyrogens
   eferent should be efferent
   thorasic should be thoracic
4. tox = poison
   immune = protection
   lytic = destroy
   onc = tumor
   lymphangi = lymph vessel

5. lymph = lymph, aden = gland, pathy = disease
   lymphadenopathy = disease of lymph glands (nodes)
   splen = spleen, rrhagia = bleeding
   splenorrhagia = bleeding from the spleen
6. (a) Nodes were removed because the main lymphatic drainage of the breast is through the axillary lymph nodes and there might be some cancer cells hidden there.
   (b) Lymph drainage from the arm was reduced due to the removal of the axillary lymph nodes, which may result in swelling.
   (c) lymphedema

CHAPTER 15

1. L (Movement of air…)
   I (Inflammation…)
   J (Accumulation of air…)
   H (Whooping cough)
   A (Suppress the cough…)
   D (Exchange of gases…)
   E (Spitting of blood …)
   C (Common cold)
   K (Swelling and fluid …)
   G (Break down mucus…)
2. VC = vital capacity
   CRD = chronic respiratory disease
   IPPB = intermittent positive-pressure breathing
   RDS = respiratory distress syndrome
   SRS = smoker's respiratory syndrome
3. (intraalveolar) intralveolar
   diaphram (diaphragm)
   (larynx) larnyx
   (pleura) plura
   emphysemia (emphysema)
4. con = dust
   capn = carbon dioxide
   rhin = nose
   ectasis = dilation
   pnea = breathing
   ptysis = spitting
   phon = voice
   rrhea = flow or discharge
   ole = little or small

anthrac = coal, coal dust
5. pneumoconiosis

CHAPTER 16

1. K (Folds in the stomach ...)
   F (Semifluid ...)
   L (Twisting of ...)
   D (An emotional disorder ...)
   H (Increase rate...)
   I (Folds in the mucosa...)
   G (Blood in the ...)
   J (Heartburn; regurgitation ...)
   B (Drugs that reduce ...)
   C (Accumulation of ...)
2. GERD = gastric esophageal reflux disease
   NVD = nausea, vomiting, diarrhea
   GI = gastrointestinal
   GB = gallbladder
   FOBT = fecal occult blood test
3. (esophageal)   esophogeal
   postpandial   (postprandial)
   glosopharyn-   (glossopharyngeal   geal)
   masetter   (masseter)
   (monoglycer-   monoglyser-
   ides)   ides
4. chole = bile, gall
   enter = small intestine
   cyst = bladder
   gingiv = gums
   hepat = liver
   orexia = appetite
   sial = saliva
   aden = gland
   ectomy = surgical removal
   emesis = vomiting
5. sialadenectomy
6. hyperemesis
7. proctalgia

CHAPTER 17

1. K (Production of ...)
   B (Amount of energy ...)
   I (Intravenous approach ...)
   E (Yellow skin ...)
   G (A state of ...)
   C (Temperature of ...)
   D (Nutrients enter ...)
   H (Deficiency of ...)
   A (Absence of ...)
   L (Inadequate food ...)
2. BED = binge eating disorder
   BMR = basal metabolic rate

HDL = high density lipoproteins
TPN = total parenteral nutrition
BMI = body mass index
3. anairobic   (anaerobic)
   asetyl-CoA   (acetyl-CoA)
   (triglycerides)   triglyserides
   (homeotherm)   homotherm
   glucogenolysis   (glycogenolysis)
4. clys = irrigation or washing out
   fruct = fruit
   pepsia = digestion
   ana = up
   lysis = to take apart
   cata = down
   mal = bad, poor
   pyr = fever, fire
   vita = life
   neo = new
5. (a) coronary artery disease
   (b) LDL or low density lipoprotein
   (c) it lodges in the capillary walls to form plaques which may eventually occlude the artery
   (d) physical activity
   (e) because fats contain over twice the number of Calories/gram; 9 C/gram for fats, 4 C/gram for carbohydrates

CHAPTER 18

1. J (Plasma)
   L (Functional unit ...)
   C (Increased amounts ...)
   M (Producing small ...)
   K (Crushing of a ...)
   B (May be caused ...)
   H (Asociated with ...)
   E (Increases production ...)
   D (Visual examination ...)
   F (Involuntary emission ...)
2. BUN = blood urea nitrogen
   ARF = acute renal failure
   GFR = glomerular filtration rate
   TUR = transurethral resection
   UTI = urinary tract infection
3. (detrusor)   detrussor
   (macula densa)   macula denca
   triagone   (trigone)
   (natriuretic)   natrietic

(albuminuria)   albuminaria
4. nephr = kidney
   cyst = bladder
   pyel = renal pelvis
   lith = calculus, stone
   azo = nitrogen
   noct = night
   peri = around
   pexy = fixation
   rrhaphy = suture
   juxta = near to
5. nocturia
6. (a) excessive ketone bodies in the blood
   (b) acidosis
   (c) metabolic
   (d) the respiratory system is compensating for the acidosis by getting rid of carbon dioxide through increased breathing rate

CHAPTER 19

1. C (Sex cells; ...)
   L (Combination estrogen ...)
   E (Abdominal pain ...)
   H (Surgical removal ...)
   G (Low sperm count)
   D (Primary reproductive ...)
   J (Synthetic progesterone)
   K (Surgical removal ...)
   B (Removal of a growth ...)
   A (Sexual intercourse ...)
2. PMS = premenstrual syndrome
   STD = sexually transmitted disease
   VD = venereal disease
   IUD = intrauterine device
   PID = pelvic inflammatory disease
3. (menarche)   menarch
   primodial   (primordial)
   pudenum   (pudendum)
   (hysterectomy)   hysterectomy
   (prostate)   prostrate
   semineferous   (seminiferous)
   (epididymis)   epidydimis
   mammry   (mammary)
   antiflexed   (anteflexed)
   (perimetrium)   parametrium
4. men = month
   fimb = fringe
   colp = vagina
   lapar = abdominal wall
   epis = vulva

orchid = testis
crypt = hidden
balan = glans
spadias = opening
ejacul = to shoot forth

5. (a) prostate-specific antigen
   (b) prostatomegaly
   (c) transurethral resection of the prostate
6. amenorrhea

CHAPTER 20

1. I (Act of giving ...)
   A (Innermost ...)
   L (Preparations that ...)
   G (Woman who has ...)
   K (An agent that causes ...)
   C (Period during which ...)
   J (Synthetic oxytocin)
   D (Good, normal childbirth)
   F (Vaginal discharge ...)
   H (Infant during ...)

2. GYN = gynecology
   HCG = human chorionic gonadotropin
   SIDS = sudden infant death syndrome
   EDD = expected delivery date
   FHR = fetal heart rate

3. (gestation)   jestation
   corion   (chorion)
   (senescence) senesance
   (zonapellu-   zonapelucida
   cida)
   clostrum   (colostrum)

4. amnio = a fetal membrane, amnion
   contra = against
   cyesi = pregnancy
   gravid = filled, pregnant
   para = to bear or bring forth
   nat = birth

5. amniorrhea = escape of the amniotic fluid
   contraceptive = diminishing the likelihood of or preventing conception
   pseudocyesis = false pregnancy
   primigravida = a woman pregnant for the first time
   nullipara = a woman who has not produced a viable offspring
   prenatal = before birth

6. (a) placenta previa
   (b) embryonic period
   (c) human chorionic gonadotropin, estrogen, progesterone

NOTES

NOTES

NOTES

NOTES